I0464571

Applied Physiology

by Frank Overton

PREFACE

This primary text-book of applied physiology follows a natural order of treatment. In each subject elementary anatomical facts are presented in a manner which impresses function rather than form, and from the form described derives the function. The facts and principles are then applied to everyday life. Anatomy and pure physiology make clear and fix hygienic points, while applied physiology lends interest to the otherwise dry facts of physiology and anatomy. From the great range of the science there are included only those subjects which are directly concerned in the growth and development of children.

The value of a primary book depends largely upon the language used. In bringing the truths within the comprehension of children, the author has made sparing use of the complex sentence. He has made the sentences short and simple in form, and logical in arrangement.

A child grasps new ideas mainly as they appeal directly to the senses. For this reason, physiological demonstrations are indispensable. Subjects for demonstrations are not given, because they cannot be performed by the children; but the teacher should make free use of the series given in the author's advanced physiology.

Cuts and diagrams are inserted where they are needed to explain the text. They are taken from the author's Applied Physiology, Intermediate Grade. Each was chosen, not for artistic effect, but because of its fitness to illustrate a point. Most of the cuts are adapted for reproduction on the blackboard.

The effects of alcohol and other narcotics are treated with special fulness. The subject is given a fair and judicial discussion, and those conclusions are presented which are universally accepted by the medical profession. But while this most important form of intemperance is singled out, it should be remembered that the breaking of any of nature's laws is also a form of intemperance, and that the whole study of applied physiology is to encourage a more healthy and a more noble and self-denying mode of life.

CONTENTS

CHAPTER I

CELLS

Our body is made of many parts. Its head thinks. Its legs carry it, and its arms and hands take hold of things. The leg cannot do the work of the arm, nor the head do the work of the hand; but each part does only its own work.

=1. The simplest animal.=--Some animals have parts like a man's; but these parts are fewer. No animal has arms or hands like a man. A fish has little fins in place of legs and arms, while a worm has not even a head, but only a body, and yet it moves. An oyster has only a body and cannot move. The simplest of all animals is very small. A thousand of them would not reach an inch. Yet each is a complete animal. It is called the ameba. It is only a lump of jelly. It can put out any part of its body like an arm and take a lump of food. This same arm can eat the food, too. It can also put out any part of its body like a leg and move by rolling the rest of its body into the leg. It can do some things better than a man can do them, for any part of its body can do all kinds of work. So the ameba grows and moves and does as it likes.

=2. Cells.=--A man's finger moves and grows something like a separate animal, but it must keep with the rest of the body. A little piece of a finger moves and grows, too. If you should look at a finger, or any other part of your body, through a microscope, you would see that it is composed of little lumps of jelly. Each little lump looks like an ameba. We call each lump a cell. The cells make up the finger.

=3. What cells do.=--Each cell acts much as an ameba does. From the blood it gets food and air and takes them in through any part of its body. It also grows and moves. But the cells are not free to do as they wish, for they are all tied together in armies by very fine strings. We call these strings connective tissue. One army of cells makes the skin, and other armies make the bones and flesh. Some armies make the fingers, and some the legs. Every part of our body is made up of armies of separate cells.

=4. The mind.=--The body is a home for the mind. The cells obey the mind. The mind pays the cells by feeding them and taking good care of them. When an army of cells is hurt, the body feels sick, and then the mind tells the whole body to rest until the cells are well again. When we study about a man's body, we learn about the separate cells in his body.

WHAT WE HAVE LEARNED

1. Our body is made up of many small parts.

2. The smallest parts are each like a little animal, and are called cells.

3. Each cell eats and grows.

4. One army of cells makes a finger and another a leg, and so on through the body.

5. The mind lives in the body.

6. The mind takes care of the cells.

CHAPTER II

OF WHAT CELLS ARE MADE

The cells of our body are made of five common things. You would know all these things if you should see them.

=5. Water.=--The first thing in the cells is water. Water is everywhere in the body. Even the teeth have water. Most of our flesh is water. Without water we should soon shrink up. Our flesh would be stiff like bone and no one could live.

=6. Albumin.=--Second, next to water, something like the white of an egg makes the most of the body. The white of an egg is albumin. When dried it is like gelatine or glue. Albumin makes the most of the solid part of each cell. Lean meat and cheese are nearly all albumin. When it is heated it becomes harder and turns white. The word albumin means white. Dry albumin is hard and tough, but in the living cells it is dissolved in water and is soft like meat. It is the only living substance in the body, and it alone gives it strength.

=7. Fat.=--Third, next to albumin, the most of the body is fat. Fat does not grow inside the cells of the body, but it fills little pockets between the cells. Fat does not give strength. It makes the body round and handsome. It also makes the cells warm and keeps them from getting hurt.

=8. Sugar.=--Fourth, sugar also is found in the body. Sugar is made out of starch. When we eat starch it changes to sugar. Starch and sugar are much alike. We eat a great deal of starch and sugar, but they are soon used in warming the body. Only a little is in the body at once.

=9. Minerals.=--Fifth, there are also some minerals in the body. When flesh is burned they are left as ashes. Salt, lime, iron, soda, and potash are all found in the body.

Everything in the body is either water, albumin, fat, sugar, or minerals. These things are also our food. We eat them mixed together in bread, meat, eggs, milk, and other foods.

=10. Life.=--Our food is not alive, but after we eat it the body makes it alive. We do not know how it does it. When the body dies we cannot put life into it again. There is life in each cell.

WHAT WE HAVE LEARNED

1. The body is made of five things: water, albumin, fat, sugar, and minerals.

2. Water is mixed with all parts of the body.

3. Albumin makes the living part of each cell.

4. Fat is in pockets between the cells. It warms the cells and keeps them from being hurt.

5. Sugar is made from starch. It warms the body.

6. The minerals in the body are salt, lime, iron, soda, and potash.

CHAPTER III

DIGESTION OF FOOD IN THE MOUTH

=11. Food of the cells.=--All the cells of the body work and wear out. They must eat and keep growing. The food of the cells is the blood. Water, albumin, fat, sugar, and minerals are in the blood. The cells eat these things and grow. All food must be one or more of these five things. Before they reach the blood, they must all be changed to a liquid. A few cells of the body are set aside to do this work of changing them. Changing food into blood is digestion.

=12. Cooking.=--Cooking begins digestion. It softens and dissolves food. It makes food taste better. Most food is unfit for use until it is cooked. Poor cooking often makes food still worse for use. Food should always be soft and taste good after cooking. Softening food by cooking saves the mouth and stomach a great deal of work. The good taste of the food makes it pleasant for them to digest it. We must cut our food into small pieces before we eat it. If we eat only a small piece at a time we shall not eat too fast. If we cut our food fine we can find any bones and other hard things, and can keep them from getting inside the body.

=13. Chewing.=--Digestion goes on in the mouth. The mouth does three things to food. First, it mixes and grinds it between the teeth.

Second, it pours water over the food through fine tubes. The water of the mouth is called the saliva. The saliva makes the food a thin paste.

Third, the saliva changes some of the starch to sugar. Starch must be all changed to sugar before it can feed the cells.

=14. Too fast eating.=--Some boys fill their mouths with food. Then they cannot chew their food and cannot mix saliva with it. They swallow their food whole, and then their stomachs have to grind it. The saliva cannot mix with the food and so it is too dry in the stomach. Then their stomachs ache, and they are sick. Eating too fast and too much makes children sick oftener than anything else.

Birds swallow their food whole, for they have no teeth. Instead, a strong gizzard inside grinds the food. We have no gizzards, and so we must grind our food with our teeth.

=15. Teeth.=--We have two kinds of teeth. The front teeth are sharp and cut the food; the back teeth are flat and rough and grind it. If you bite nuts or other hard things you may break off a little piece of a tooth. Then the tooth may decay and ache.

After you eat, some food will sometimes stick to the teeth. Then it may decay and make your breath smell bad. After each meal always pick the teeth with a wooden toothpick. Your teeth will also get dirty and become stained unless you clean them. Always brush your teeth with water every morning. This will also keep them from decaying.

=16. Swallowing.=--When food has been chewed and mixed with saliva until it is a paste, it is ready to be swallowed. The tongue pushes the food into a bag just back of the mouth. We call the bag the pharynx. Then the pharynx squeezes it down a long tube and into the stomach. The nose and windpipe also open into this bag, but both are closed by little doors while we swallow. We cannot breathe while we swallow. If the doors are not shut tightly, some food gets into the windpipe and chokes us.

WHAT WE HAVE LEARNED

1. We eat to feed the cells of the body.

2. All food must be made into blood.

3. Changing food to blood is digestion.

4. Cooking softens food and makes it taste good.

5. Food is ground fine in the mouth, and mixed with saliva to form a paste. Some of its starch is changed to sugar.

6. If food is only half chewed the stomach has to grind it.

7. When we swallow, the tongue pushes the food into a bag back of the mouth and the bag squeezes it down a long tube to the stomach.

CHAPTER IV

DIGESTION IN THE STOMACH

=17. The stomach.=--When food is swallowed it goes to the stomach. The stomach is a thin bag. In a man it holds about three pints. Like the mouth, it does three things to the food.

First, the stomach gently stirs and mixes the food.

Second, it pours a fluid over the food. This fluid is called the gastric juice.

The gastric juice is sour and bitter.

Third, the gastric juice changes some of the albumin of food to a liquid form.

If the mouth has done its work well, the stomach does its work easily and we do not know it. But if the mouth has eaten food too fast and has not chewed it well, then the stomach must do the work of the mouth too. In that case it gets tired and aches.

=18. The intestine.=--The food stays in the stomach only a little while. All the time a little keeps trickling into a long coil of tube. This tube is called the intestine or the bowels. Three or four hours after a hearty meal the stomach is empty. Some of the food has been changed to a liquid, but most of it has only been ground to smaller pieces, and mixed with a great deal of water. Now it all must be changed to a liquid.

=19. What the intestine does.=--Like the mouth and stomach, the intestine does three things.

First, it mixes the food and makes it pass down the tube.

Second, two sets of cells behind the stomach make two liquids and pour them into the intestine. One set of cells is the sweetbread, or pancreas, and its liquid is the pancreatic juice. The other is the liver and its fluid is the bile.

Third, the pancreatic juice makes three changes in food. First, like the mouth, it changes starch to sugar. Second, like the stomach, it makes albumin a liquid. Third, it divides fat into fine drops. These drops then mix with water and do not float on its top.

=20. Bile.=--The bile is yellow and bitter. It helps the pancreatic juice do its work. It also helps to keep the inside of the intestine clean.

=21. Digestion of water and minerals.=--Water and the mineral parts of food do not need to be changed at all, but can become part of the blood just as they are. Seeds and husks and tough strings of flesh all pass the length of the intestine and are not changed.

=22. How food gets into the blood.=--By the time food is half way down the intestine it is mostly liquid and ready to become part of the blood. This liquid soaks through the sides of the intestine and into the blood tubes. At last the food reaches the end of the intestine. Most of its liquid has then soaked into the blood tubes and only some solid waste is left.

=23. Work of the liver.=--The food is now in the blood, but has not become a part of it. It is carried to the liver. There the liver changes the food to good blood, and then the blood hurries on and feeds the cells of the body. Spoiled food may be swallowed and taken into the blood with the good food. The liver takes out the poisons and sends them back again with the bile. The liver keeps us from getting poisoned.

=24. Bad food.=--Sometimes the stomach and intestine cannot digest the food. They cannot digest green apples, but they try hard to do so. They stir the apples faster and faster until there is a great pain. Sometimes the stomach throws up the food and then the pain and sickness stop. Spoiled food makes us sick in the same way.

=25. Too fast eating.=--When the food stays too long in the stomach or intestine it sours, or decays, just as it does outside of the body. This makes us very sick. When we eat too much, or when we do not chew the food to small pieces, the stomach may be a long time in digesting the food. Then it may become sour and make us sick.

=26. Biliousness.=--When the food is poor or becomes sour, it is poorly digested. Then the liver has more work to do, and does not change the food to blood as it should. It also lets some of the sour poisons pass by it. These poison the whole body and make the head ache. We call this biliousness. The tongue is then covered with a white or yellow coat and the mouth tastes bad.

These are signs of sickness. The stomach and liver are out of order.

=27. Rules for eating.=--If we eat as we should, our stomach will digest its food. We must follow three rules.

First, we must chew the food in the mouth until all the lumps are fine. Then the food will be ready for the stomach.

Second, we must eat slowly. If we eat fast we cannot chew the food well. The stomach cannot take care of food if it comes too fast. We must swallow all of one mouthful before we put another into the mouth.

Third, we must eat only at meal times. The stomach needs a rest. Even a little candy, or apples, or nuts will keep the stomach at work, and tire it out. A child needs to eat more often than his father. So, besides his meals, he should have something to eat in the middle of the morning and some more in the afternoon. But he should not be eating at all hours. He ought not to eat little bits just before dinner, for that spoils his meal.

WHAT WE HAVE LEARNED

1. The stomach and intestine stir and rub the food, and mix it with juices.

2. The juices change albumin to a liquid, and starch to sugar. They also change fat to the form of tiny drops.

3. The digested food soaks through the sides of the intestine into the blood tubes.

4. The blood carries the food to the liver.

5. The liver changes food to blood.

6. Blood goes to all parts of the body and feeds the cells.

7. The liver keeps poisons from getting into the blood.

8. Water and minerals become a part of the blood without being digested.

9. When food is not well digested, the liver cannot make it into good blood. This makes us bilious.

10. If food is not soon digested it sours and decays. This makes us sick.

11. We can make food digest quickly by chewing it well and eating slowly.

CHAPTER V

FOODS

=28. Kinds of food.=--The cells of the body need water, albumin, fat, sugar, and minerals for food. We sometimes eat sugar alone, and we drink pure water. But most of our food is a mixture of all five kinds of food. Food comes from animals and plants.

=29. Milk=.--Milk is the best food known. It contains just enough water, albumin, fat, sugar, and minerals. Babies and young mammals live on milk alone. A man can live upon four quarts of milk a day. In sickness, milk is the very best food for men, as well as for babies.

The albumin of milk becomes hard when the milk sours. This makes cheese. The fat of milk rises to the top. We call it cream. When cream is churned, the pure fat comes together in a lump. Pure fat of milk is called butter. Cheese and butter are both good foods.

=30. Eggs.=--Eggs are also good food. The white of an egg is almost pure albumin. The yolk is albumin and fat. Eggs have no starch or sugar. They are not a perfect food, for some sugar must be eaten. But they can be quickly digested and they produce a great deal of strength.

=31. Meat.=--Meat contains albumin and fat, but no sugar. Fish, oysters, and clams are like meat. They all make good food. Boys and girls should eat milk, eggs, and meat. These foods are the best to give strength to the body. Nearly all food from animals is more quickly digested and gives more strength than food from plants.

=32. Bread.=--White bread is a food made from wheat. The wheat is ground to flour. Flour is mixed with water, and yeast is added. The yeast makes a gas, and the gas puffs up the wet flour and makes it full of holes. The holes make the bread light. Then bread is baked. Rye or corn meal makes good bread. Cake, biscuit, and pancakes are much like bread. Sometimes in place of yeast, baking powder is used to make the bread or cake light.

=33. Meal.=--Oatmeal, corn meal, and cracked wheat and rice are sometimes boiled, and eaten with milk. Bread, biscuit, oatmeal, and corn meal are made from grain. All are very much alike. The cooking makes them look and taste different, but yet they are nearly the same.

=34. Why we need grain food.=--All kinds of grain have much albumin, but only a little fat. But all have a great deal of starch. By digestion the starch becomes sugar. Grain is a good food because it has starch or sugar. Animal foods have no sugar, so we eat grain food with them. The two together make the most nourishing food. Potatoes have a great deal of starch and only a little albumin. They also are good food with meat.

A person cannot live well upon plant food alone, for it has too much starch and sugar, and too little albumin and fat. We need nearly equal parts of albumin, fat, and sugar. A mixture of bread, meat, eggs, vegetables, and milk makes the best food.

=35. Fruit.=--Fruit, like apples, peaches, and plums all have sugar. They taste good, and give us an appetite for other kinds of food. They have little albumin or fat.

=36. Salt.=--There is enough mineral matter in all food, and we do not have to eat iron or lime or soda. But we do need some more salt. Even animals need salt. Salt makes food taste good, and helps its digestion.

[Illustration: =People are made sick by drinking water from such a well.=]

=37. Water.=--Water is also a food, for it forms the most of our bodies. All food has water. Even dry crackers contain it.

=38. Pure water.=--Water in a well runs through the dirty earth, and yet is clear and pure. This is because sand holds back the dirt. But sometimes slops from the house, and water from the barn yard, soak through the soil until the sand is full. Then the well water will be dirty and poisonous. People are often made sick by drinking such water. In cities the dirt fills all the soil and spoils the water. So the water must be brought from the country in large pipes.

Water in lead pipes takes up some of the lead. Lead is a poison. You should let the water run off from a pipe a little while before you use it. Good water is clear and has no smell or taste. Dirty or yellow water, or water with a taste or smell, is not fit for use.

=39. Tea and coffee.=--Tea and coffee are steeped in water and used as a drink. The drink is the water. The tea and coffee are neither food nor drink. They cause the cells of the body to do more work, and at the same time they take away the feeling of being tired. They do not give strength to the body, but are like a whip and make the body work harder.

=40. The appetite.=--When we have so many kinds of food, what kind is best for us? The taste of food tells us the kind of food to eat. Bread and meat, and such plain foods, always taste good, and we never get tired of them. Sugar tastes good until we get enough. Any more makes us sick. More than enough sugar or starch is found in bread and potatoes.

If we can eat food day after day, without getting tired of it, the food is good for us. If we get tired of its taste, either the food is not good for us or we are eating too much. Bad tasting or bad smelling food is always dangerous.

We can tell how much food to eat by our hunger or appetite. We can always feel when we have enough. Then is the time to stop.

Sometimes we eat plain bread and meat until we have enough, and then sweet cake or pie is brought in. Then we have a false appetite for sweet things. If the sweet things had not made a false hunger, we should have had enough to eat. But the false appetite makes us want more, and so we eat too much, and sometimes get sick from it.

=41. Intemperance.=--Eating for the sake of a false appetite is intemperance. Drinking strong drink for the sake of its taste is a common form of intemperance. But eating too much preserves, pie, and candy is intemperance too, and can do a great deal of harm. A little pie, or pudding, or candy, is good, because we can eat our sugar as well that way as in bread. But we should eat only a little.

=42. Food and Diseases.=--If our food is dirty or is handled with dirty hands, or is put into dirty dishes, there may be disease germs in it. Our food should always be clean, and we should have our hands clean when we handle it or eat it.

Storekeepers sometimes keep fruit and vegetables out of doors where street dust may blow upon it. This dust is often full of disease germs. Flies may also bring disease germs to the food. If food is kept where dust and flies can get at it, we ought not to buy it.

WHAT WE HAVE LEARNED

1. Food is a mixture of water, albumin, fat, starch or sugar, and minerals.

2. Animal foods, like milk, eggs, and meat, have albumin and fat in the best form.

3. Plant food has albumin and fat, but it has very much starch or sugar. So, taken together with animal food, it makes a complete food.

4. Lime, iron, soda, and salt are found in all foods, but we must add a little more salt to food.

5. Water is found in all food, but we must drink some besides.

6. Dirty water, or water with a taste or smell, is not fit for use.

7. Taste tells us what kind of food to use.

8. Hunger, or the appetite, tells us how much food to use.

9. There can be a false hunger for sweet things. This may lead us to eat too much.

10. Eating too much of sweet things is one form of intemperance.

CHAPTER VI

TOBACCO

=43. Harmful eating.=--Men often eat for the fun of eating, and sometimes they eat harmful things. They chew tobacco and drink strong drinks, because they like their taste, just as a child eats candy.

=44. Tobacco.=--Men have always drunk strong drink. Within the last four hundred years, men have learned another way to please a wrong taste. When Columbus discovered America, the Indians were using tobacco. They taught the Spaniards how to smoke it, and since then almost the whole world has used it.

Tobacco is the leaf of a tall plant. It needs a better soil than any other crop. It takes the richness from the ground, and spoils it for other crops.

=45. Nicotine.=--About 1/30 of each tobacco leaf is a strong poison. This poison is called nicotine. A drop or two of it, or as much of it as is in a strong cigar, will kill a man. It gives the tobacco its smell and taste. Men use tobacco for the sake of a poison.

=46. Why men use tobacco.=--Men give queer reasons for using tobacco. One smokes for its company, another because he is with company. One smokes to make his brain think better, and another to keep himself from thinking. Some use tobacco to help digest their food, and others use it to keep themselves from eating so much. Boys smoke to make themselves look like men. The real reason for using tobacco is that men learn to like its taste, and do not care if it harms them.

=47. Spitting.=--Tobacco in any form makes the saliva flow. Men do not dare swallow it, for it makes them sick. So they spit it out. No one likes to see this. It is a dirty and filthy habit. Besides, the saliva is lost, and cannot help digest food.

Tobacco stains the teeth brown. You can always tell a tobacco chewer by his teeth. His breath will smell of tobacco, and even his clothes are offensive to the nose.

=48. Tobacco lessens strength.=--Tobacco always makes a person sick at the stomach, at first. After a while, he becomes used to it, and an ordinary chew or smoke does not make him sick. But a large chew or smoke will always make him sick again. When a person is sick from tobacco he is very weak. Even if he is not sick, the tobacco poisons his muscles and makes his strength less. When a man trains for a hard race he never uses tobacco.

=49. Tobacco hinders digestion.=--Tobacco and its smoke both have a burning taste. This makes the throat sore, and causes a cough. Tobacco does not help the stomach to digest food. Smokers and chewers often have headaches and coated tongues. These are signs of a poor digestion.

=50. Effect upon the young.=--Tobacco is more harmful to boys than to men. If boys smoke they cannot run fast or long. They cannot work hard with their brains or hands. They do not grow fast, and are liable to have weak hearts.

=51. Tobacco harms others.=--Many persons do not like the smell of tobacco, and no one likes the spit. No one should use it in the presence of others. The tobacco user's pleasure should not spoil the comfort and happiness of others.

=52. Snuff.=--Powdered tobacco is called snuff. Snuff causes sneezing. No one should harm the nose and the whole body for the pleasure of a sneeze. Years ago snuff was used much more than it is now.

=53. Chewing.=--Chewing tobacco is the most poisonous way of using it, for it keeps most of the nicotine in the mouth. Chewing will make any one very sick, unless he spits out all the saliva.

=54. Smoking.=--Men smoke pipes, cigars, and cigarettes. The smoke has nicotine, and is poisonous. Pipe stems get dirty and full of nicotine. After a while they smell bad and are very poisonous. An old smoker's pipe will make a young smoker sick.

=55. Cigarettes.=--Cigars are not so poisonous as a pipe, for more of the nicotine is burned up. Cigarettes are often made of weak tobacco. A cigarette does not contain so much tobacco as a cigar. Hence a cigarette does not cost much. It can be smoked in a hurry. It does not make a boy so sick as cigars do. Boys and men use a great many cigarettes where they would not touch a cigar. This makes the use of cigarettes the most dangerous form of smoking. Selling cigarettes to young boys is forbidden by law.

=56. Habit.=--When men have used tobacco for some time, they like it and feel bad without it. So they get into the habit of using it, and find it hard to stop. The tobacco seems to help them, but it does not do so. It cheats men, and they do not know it.

=57. Chewing gum.=--Chewing gum is made from pitch or paraffin, for these substances will not dissolve in the mouth. The gum is flavored with sugar and spices. The gum and its flavors are not harmful in themselves, and yet chewing them is harmful. Chewing makes a great deal of saliva flow. All this saliva is wasted, and when we eat our meals we may have too little. Then our food will not digest well, but we shall have dyspepsia and headaches.

By pulling and handling the gum while chewing it, you may get some poisonous dirt into your mouth, and make yourself very sick.

Even if your gum should not harm you, there is a good reason for letting it alone. When you are chewing gum, you look as if you were chewing tobacco. No one likes to see a boy or girl even appearing to chew tobacco. If you form a habit of chewing gum you will be more likely to chew tobacco when you are grown.

WHAT WE HAVE LEARNED

1. Men use tobacco for the sake of its nicotine. Nicotine is a very strong poison.

2. Tobacco causes a man to waste his saliva.

3. Tobacco makes the mouth dry.

4. Tobacco hinders digestion.

5. Tobacco stains the teeth, and makes the breath smell bad.

6. Tobacco makes a person sick at the stomach.

7. Tobacco weakens the muscles.

8. Tobacco is more harmful to the young than to grown persons.

9. Chewing is the worst form of using tobacco.

10. Smoking cigarettes is the worst form of smoking.

CHAPTER VII

FERMENTATION

=58. Souring of fruit.=--When a little fruit is set away in a warm place for a day or two it sours or ferments. Anything sweet will do the same thing. Little bubbles rise up through the juice and a foam comes on top. Then the juice has a sharp taste or is sour. Canned and preserved fruit becomes sour soon after the jar is opened, and cider soon turns to vinegar. All fruit juice does this even in cold weather. But in cold weather it keeps for a longer time.

=59. Preserving fruit.=--If your mother wishes to keep fruit all winter she boils it and at once puts it into tight jars. This shuts out the air and then the fruit keeps good all winter. Boiling kills all living things, and no more can get in through the tight jars. Does a living thing have anything to do with making the fruit juice turn sour?

=60. Yeast.=--Yeast will make all sweet things ferment. Bakers make yeast grow in bread sponge. Yeast is alive. It is made of millions of tiny round cells. New cells sprout out from the side of the old cells like young lilies on an old lily bulb. Soon each new cell breaks off and lives all by itself. In a single night enough new cells will form to fill the whole loaf of bread.

=61. How yeast makes alcohol.=--Yeast will grow only where sugar is. When it has grown for some time there is no more sugar, and instead of a sweet taste there is a sharp or sour taste. The yeast has changed the sugar to alcohol. All alcohol is made from sugar by yeast.

The seeds of the yeast plant are everywhere in the air. Some are on the skins of fruit and so are found in the juice when it is squeezed out. There they begin to grow at once and soon change the sugar to alcohol. They do this by taking a gas away from the sugar. The gas rises in little bubbles, and makes a froth upon the top of the juice. Boiling kills the yeast plant. If the juice is at once put into tight jars no new yeast plants can get in, and so the juice keeps.

=62. Vinegar.=--Sometimes fruit juice turns sour. The sourness is due to vinegar. Besides yeast, other little living plants fall into the juice and turn the sugar to vinegar. But if there is much alcohol in the juice, the vinegar plants will not grow.

=63. Yeast in bread.=--Growing yeast plants always make alcohol. They change some of the sugar of bread dough to alcohol and a gas. The gas bubbles through the bread and makes it light. When bread is baked, the heat of the oven drives off the alcohol, and so we do not eat any in bread.

=64. Alcohol.=--Alcohol is a clear liquid and looks like water. It has a sharp taste and smell. It burns very easily and makes a very hot flame. Its smoke cannot be seen, and its flame will not make anything black, as a match flame will do.

=65. Use of alcohol.=--Alcohol will dissolve more things than water will dissolve. It is used to dissolve drugs, varnishes, perfumery, and many other things. It will dissolve even oil and fat. Tailors clean grease spots from clothes with it. It takes water away from flesh and makes it dry, hard, and tough. It will keep anything from rotting. In museums we pour alcohol over pieces of flesh or plants in glass jars. Then they will keep and we can look at them at any time. Thus alcohol is a very useful thing, and we could hardly do without it.

=66. Strong drink.=--Some men use alcohol in a wrong way. They swallow it as a drink. But men cannot drink pure alcohol, for it would burn their mouths. They always drink it mixed with some water. Alcohol in water is called strong drink.

=67. Why men use strong drink.=--Some men take strong drink to make themselves warm, and some to make themselves cool. Some drink to keep themselves awake, and some to make themselves sleep. Some drink to keep themselves still, and some to make themselves stir around faster. Men use strong drink really because it seems to make them feel strong for a while. It does not make them stronger, but it harms the body and the mind. Its alcohol does the harm.

WHAT WE HAVE LEARNED

1. Sugar in fruit or in water turns to alcohol or vinegar, and a gas.

2. The change to alcohol is caused by the cells of the yeast plant.

3. The change to vinegar is caused by another small plant.

4. Boiling fruit juice kills the yeast plants and then the juice will keep without change.

5. Alcohol looks like water. It has a sharp and burning taste.

6. Alcohol takes water from flesh and hardens it.

7. Alcohol burns with a great heat and no smoke.

8. Alcohol is used to dissolve things, and to keep things from spoiling.

9. Alcohol in water forms strong drink.

CHAPTER VIII

KINDS OF STRONG DRINK

=68. Wine.=--All strong drink is alcohol and water. There may be other things to give it taste, but alcohol and water are always in it. No strong drink is over one half alcohol.

In olden times wine was the only strong drink. Men used to crush out the juice of grapes and let it ferment. This made wine. But very often they used the juice before it fermented. Then it had no alcohol and could do no harm, but was a good food. We read of wine in the Bible. Some of it was fresh fruit juice.

In wine, the sugar is changed to alcohol. The rest of the juice stays the same. All wine is made by the yeast plant growing in fruit juice. No yeast is put in, for there is always enough on the outside of the fruit. Wine is about one tenth alcohol.

=69. Homemade wine.=--Cider is a kind of wine. It is made from apple juice. It has alcohol a day or two after it is made. All homemade wines have alcohol. Any of them can make a person drunk. Using weak homemade wine and cider often makes an appetite for stronger drinks. The alcohol in any of them is enough to harm the body.

=70. Beer.=--After man had made wine for a long time, some one found out how to cultivate yeast. Then men could make sugar and water ferment whenever they wanted to. So men boiled grain to take out its sugar. Then they poured off the liquor and added yeast and let it ferment. This made beer and ale. Now millions of bushels of grain are used every year in making beer. Men call beer a light drink. But it has alcohol and is a strong drink, and can make men drunk.

=71. Root beer.=--Some persons boil roots and herbs, and add molasses and yeast. Then the liquid ferments and becomes root beer. They say "it has no alcohol, for we made it." But it does have alcohol, for yeast always makes alcohol. Some ginger ale is made by putting yeast in sweetened ginger water. It has alcohol, too.

=72. Distillation.=--Boiling water turns to vapor or steam and goes off in the air. When the vapor is cooled, you can see the water again. It often cools on the window and makes little streams of water. You can catch the steam in a tube. If you keep the tube cool, the steam will turn to water in the tube. This process is called distillation.

[Illustration: =A glass of whisky contains so much alcohol.=]

Boiling alcohol also passes off into the air as vapor. When the vapor is cooled, it becomes liquid again. Alcohol boils with less heat than water. When alcohol in water is heated, the alcohol boils first. So the vapor has more alcohol than the water. When the vapor is cooled, the liquid has more alcohol than it had at first. When the liquid is distilled again it has more alcohol yet. Pure alcohol can be made in this way.

=73. Whisky.=--Distilling wine or strong beer makes whisky and brandy. Whisky is one half alcohol. It is more harmful than wine or beer.

=74. Habit.=--Some strong drinks have only a little alcohol and some have a great deal. No one begins to drink the strong liquors. He begins with wine or beer. When he has once learned, he has a hard time to stop drinking. It is dangerous to drink even weak drinks.

=75. Strong drink and thirst.=--When a man is thirsty, water will satisfy him but strong drink will not. Sometimes the mouth is dry and dirty and then a man feels thirsty. Rinsing the mouth with water, and rubbing the tongue and teeth clean will help the dryness and stop the thirst. At any rate, strong drink will only make the mouth dryer.

Some men drink only when they are tired. Then a cup of strong and hot tea or coffee will make them feel much better than a glass of strong drink, and will not harm them so much.

When strong drink is swallowed, its alcohol takes water from the mouth. When your mouth is dry, you feel thirsty. Strong drink makes the mouth dry, and so a drink makes a man more thirsty. The alcohol also makes the mouth smart. Men need another drink to cool the mouth after the first one. So one drink leads to another. All the while a person drinks water with the alcohol until he has too much water. But his mouth is dry and he feels as thirsty as ever.

=76. Effect of alcohol upon the stomach.=--When strong drink is swallowed it makes the stomach smart just as it does the mouth. So the stomach feels warm, but it is really no warmer. This harms the stomach and keeps it from working well.

Alcohol also keeps the gastric juice from changing albumin to a liquid. Alcohol keeps flesh from decaying in a museum. In the same way it may hinder the digestion of food in the stomach.

When alcohol is used for only a short time, the stomach can get well; but if it is used for months and years, the stomach will stay weak. Then the drinker can hardly eat at all.

=77. What becomes of alcohol.=--In the stomach a great deal of gastric juice is mixed with the alcohol. So it is very weak when it reaches the intestine. Alcohol needs only a little digesting. It soon soaks into the blood from the intestine along with the other food. The blood flows fast and washes the alcohol away as soon as it leaves the intestine. Too little gets into the blood at once to harm it much.

Alcohol goes to the liver, and is there destroyed; but it still does great harm. The liver has to attend to the alcohol, and so it does not change the food to good blood, and it does not take all the poisons out of the blood. Then the whole body becomes weak and sick. Alcohol hurts the liver first, and more than other parts of the body. On this account, drinkers often have bilious attacks and stomach troubles.

=78. Bitters.=--Many medicines are made by dissolving drugs in alcohol. In taking a strong medicine, we use only a few drops, and so do not get much alcohol. Some kinds of medicines must be taken in large doses. Bitters are weak medicines, and must be taken by the tablespoonful. A tablespoonful of the medicine has more alcohol than a large drink of whisky. The bitters seem to make a person feel well, but it is because he is taking a large amount of strong drink.

Jamaica Ginger is only common ginger dissolved in alcohol. It, too, is a form of strong drink.

=79. Strong drink as medicine.=--People sometimes keep whisky or brandy in the house to give for colds or other slight forms of sickness. A drink of hot coffee does more good than the strong drink, and has none of its dangers.

By using whisky or brandy for medicine, children learn to believe in strong drink, and so they will be likely to use it when they grow up. This reason alone ought to keep any one from giving it to a child.

=80. Alcohol in cooking.=--In making bread, alcohol is formed in the dough by the yeast. When the bread is baked, all the alcohol is driven off by the heat, and so we do not eat any.

Sometimes brandy or wine is put into desserts. If it is put in after the dessert is cooked, we shall get as much alcohol as if we had drunk it. If the liquor is put in before cooking, the heat will drive off the alcohol but the flavor of the liquor will remain. The flavor will do no harm in itself, but people will learn its taste, and from it may learn to like the strong drink itself. The alcohol in bread has no special flavor and does not leave any taste behind. So we cannot learn to like strong drink by eating bread.

WHAT WE HAVE LEARNED

1. Fruit juice makes wine or cider.

2. All kinds of wine contain alcohol.

3. When the liquid from boiled grain has fermented, it becomes beer, or ale.

4. By boiling wine or beer, and cooling the vapor, distilled drinks like whisky are made. They are one half alcohol.

5. Water will satisfy a real thirst. Strong drink will not.

6. Alcohol keeps the stomach from digesting food.

7. Alcohol soaks into the blood tubes and goes to the liver.

8. The liver destroys the alcohol, but is hurt in doing it.

CHAPTER IX

THE BLOOD

=81. Blood.=--After food becomes blood, it goes to every part of the body to feed the cells. Even a pin prick anywhere in the body draws blood. The blood makes the skin pink. There are five or six quarts of blood in a man's body. This is about 1/13 of his body.

Blood looks like a red liquid. But if you look at it through a strong microscope, it looks like water, and millions of little red cells. These cells carry air through the body. They make the blood look red. There are also a smaller number of white cells. Blood is made of red cells, white cells, and a liquid.

=82. The liquid in blood.=--The liquid part of the blood is albumin, and water, with a little fat, sugar, and minerals. It is food and drink for the cells of the body. When blood is drawn from the body it soon becomes like jelly. We call the jelly a clot. When you cut your finger, a clot forms in the cut and plugs up the bleeding place. If it did not, the blood would all run out of the body and we should die.

=83. The heart.=--The blood is held in tubes. A pump inside the body keeps it always moving. This pump is called the heart. The heart is a bag of muscle with thick sides. It is about as large as your fist. When it is full, it has the power to make itself smaller, and so it squeezes the blood out through a tube. We can feel each squeeze as a heart-beat. You can find the heart-beat just to the left of the middle of the body about two hand-breadths below the neck.

=84. The heart-beat.=--A man's heart beats about seventy times each minute. Boys' and girls' hearts beat much faster. Running or hard work of any kind makes the heart beat faster yet. Your heart will keep on beating until you die. It does not seem to rest at all, yet it works only while you feel it beat. Between each beat it rests while the blood is filling it again. So it really rests one half of the time.

=85. Arteries.=--The heart pumps the blood through a single tube. This tube opens into smaller tubes. These open into still smaller ones. You must use a strong microscope to see the finest blood tubes. The tubes reach every part of the body, and carry blood to its cells. They are called arteries. At each heart-beat a wave of blood can be felt in an artery. This wave is the pulse. It can be felt in the wrist, temples, and other places. By the pulse we can tell how often and how strongly the heart is beating.

=86. Capillaries.=--The smallest arteries divide into a fine network of small tubes. These tubes are the capillaries. They lie around every cell of the body.

Their sides are very thin. As the blood flows through them, some of it soaks through the sides of the tubes. Blood contains all kinds of food for the cells. Each cell is always wet with food and can eat it at any time. The cells are like the tiny animal, the ameba, and can take in the food by any part of their bodies. The cells are better off than the ameba, for their food is brought to them. They pay the body for their food by working for it.

=87. Veins.=--The capillaries come together again to form large tubes. These tubes are called veins. Only a little of the blood goes through the sides of a capillary. The rest flows on into the veins. The veins unite to form two large tubes. These two tubes open into the heart.

=88. How the blood flows.=--The blood is pumped out of the heart, through the arteries to the capillaries. There some goes out to the cells. The rest flows into the veins and goes back to the heart. All the blood in the body passes through the heart every two minutes. It takes only twenty seconds for a drop of blood to go from the heart to the toes and back again. The arteries are deep in the flesh, but some of the large veins can be seen upon the back of the hands.

=89. Bleeding.=--If a large artery or vein is cut there is a great deal of bleeding. You can always stop a cut from bleeding by holding it fast between the hands. Do not be afraid of the blood when you see any one bleeding, but hold the sides of the cut tightly with both of your hands. This will stop any bleeding until help comes. You may keep a person from bleeding to death by doing this when other persons are afraid of the blood.

=90. Healing cuts.=--When your flesh is cut it soon grows together again. The work of the little white cells in the blood is to help heal cuts and wounds and bruises. These cells are like little amebas in the blood. They keep moving around with the blood, and now and then burrow outside the capillaries to see if all is well. If they find a cut, hundreds and thousands rush to the spot at once. Some eat up any specks of dirt on the cut. Others fit themselves into the sides of the cut and grow long and slender, like strings, and so bind the two edges of the cut together. In this way all cuts are healed.

=91. The white blood cells kill disease germs.=--There are tiny living beings everywhere in the air, and soil, and water. Some of them can grow inside a man and make him sick. These tiny things are called disease germs. One kind gives a man typhoid fever, and another diphtheria. Another kind grows on cuts, and sometimes makes them very sore. The white cells of the blood are always watching for these enemies, like a cat hunting mice, and when they find them they at once try to kill them. But sometimes the white blood cells get killed. Then they look like cream in the cut. We call this creamy liquid matter or pus, and say "We have caught cold in the cut." In most pricks and cuts the white cells of the blood can kill all these enemies and also heal the cut.

=92. Catching cold.=--Sometimes the cold air blows on our head and hurts the cells of the nose. If there are disease germs in the air, they may grow in the injured part of the nose and make us have a "cold in the head." Then the white blood cells gather at the spot so as to kill the disease germs. Also the arteries bring a great deal of blood to the nose so as to heal the injured parts. Some of the white blood cells and the liquid from the blood run out, and we have to blow the nose. The white blood cells help to make us well whenever we catch a cold or other kind of sickness.

=93. Red blood cells.=--The red blood cells are like tiny flat plates. They float in the liquid part of the blood and make the blood look red. They carry air from the lungs to the cells of every part of the body, and thus help all the cells to breathe.

=94. Why the heart beats hard when we run.=--When we work hard, the cells of our bodies need a great deal of food. So the heart beats much harder, and sends them much more blood. We can feel our heart beat when we run hard.

When the cells work they get more blood in another way. The arteries become larger and hold more blood. Then the part looks red and feels warm. Thus your face gets red when you run hard. This is because your heart and arteries bring more blood to feed the working cells.

=95. Need of a strong heart.=--The heart must keep sending blood to feed the cells. If it should stop for only a little while, the cells would starve to death and we should die. We need strong hearts. When we work very hard for a long time, the heart gets tired. Then the cells do not get enough food and we feel weak all over. Boys ought not to run and lift till they are tired out, for this hurts their hearts.

=96. What alcohol does to the blood.=--Alcohol hinders the digestion of food. Then too little food will reach the blood, and so the cells of the body will get too little. Alcohol does not add strength to the body, but it takes it away. It seems to make men stronger, for it takes away their tired feelings. But it makes them really weaker, for it harms the blood.

=97. How alcohol affects the heart.=--Alcohol at first makes the heart beat more strongly and quickly, but it tires it out and makes it weaker. Then the heart pumps too little blood to the rest of the body, and a man is weaker all over.

If a drinker tries to run or work hard, his heart may not pump enough food to the working cells of his arms and legs. Strong drink takes away a man's strength and makes him less able to endure a long strain.

=98. How alcohol harms the arteries.=--Alcohol causes the arteries to become larger and to carry more blood. Then the face will be red and the skin will become warm. This makes a person feel well, and he seems to be helped. His blood seems to be flowing faster because his face is red. But really it is flowing slower.

When the arteries have been made large very often, they stay large all the time. A drinker's nose is often red from this cause.

Alcohol sometimes causes the arteries to become hard, and even to change to a kind of bone. Then they cannot change their size to carry just so much blood as each part needs.

=99. How tobacco affects the heart.=--Tobacco weakens all the body, but it harms the heart more than the rest. It often makes the heart beat slowly at one time and fast at another. It weakens the heart and keeps it from working harder when the working cells need more food. A smoker gets out of breath quickly. He cannot run far or work very hard. Chewing is a still more harmful form of using tobacco. When men train for a game or a race they never use tobacco.

Boys are not so strong as men, and so tobacco is more hurtful to them. Boys are harmed by tobacco far more than men. Cigarette smoke harms their stomachs and keeps food from their blood. If boys smoke, they become pale and weak. The poisonous smoke weakens the heart, and they cannot run or work so hard as they should. Even if a father uses tobacco, he should not allow his boys to use it.

WHAT WE HAVE LEARNED

1. Blood is a liquid. It contains many round red cells and a few white cells.

2. Blood contains all kinds of food for the cells of the body.

3. The blood is kept moving by the heart.

4. The heart pumps or beats about seventy times a minute.

5. The blood flows through arteries to all parts of the body.

6. The arteries open into the capillaries. Capillaries make a network around each cell of the body.

7. Some of the liquid parts of the blood go out through the sides of the capillaries and become food for the cells of the body.

8. From the capillaries the blood flows into the veins and back to the heart.

9. Bleeding can be stopped by holding the cut tightly between the hands.

10. The white blood cells grow into the sides of cuts, and so heal them. They also guard the body against the seeds of many diseases.

11. The red blood cells carry air to the cells of the body.

12. Alcohol weakens the heart and arteries.

13. Tobacco harms the heart.

CHAPTER X

BREATHING, HEAT, AND CLOTHING

=100. The lungs.=--Our food becomes blood and feeds the cells of our body, but we grow only a little heavier. What becomes of the food?

Besides food, air is always getting into our bodies. In breathing, air passes through the nose into a tube in the neck. This tube is called the windpipe. You can feel it as a pile of hard rings in the front part of the neck. The windpipe divides into many branches. At the end of its smallest branches are little bags or sacs. The branches and the sacs make the two lungs. So a lung is a soft and spongy piece of flesh, and can be blown up like a rubber bag. A frog's lung is a single, thin bag, about half an inch across it. Each little sac of a man's lung is like a tiny frog's lung.

=101. The diaphragm.=--The lungs fill the upper part of the body just below the neck. They are covered by the bony ribs, and rest upon a broad muscle. This muscle is called the diaphragm. It divides the inside of the body into two parts. The upper part is the chest, and holds the heart and lungs. The lower part is the abdomen, and holds the stomach, intestine, and liver, and a few other parts.

=102. Breathing.=--When the diaphragm lowers itself, or the ribs are raised, the chest is made larger. Then the air rushes through the nose and swells out the lungs to the size of the chest. This is taking a breath. Then the chest becomes smaller again, and blows the air out. A man breathes about eighteen times a minute. He does not seem to rest in breathing, but as he works only when he takes in breath, he rests one half of the time.

=103. How air gets into the blood.=--After the blood has been around the body through the arteries and capillaries and veins, the heart sends every drop to the lungs before it sends it out to feed the cells again. The blood flows through little capillaries upon the sides of the air sacs. There the red blood cells take up some of the air, and carry it with them. When they have a load of air, they become of a brighter red color. The blood in the arteries on its way to the cells is bright red.

=104. How the cells get air.=--When the blood reaches the capillaries around the cells of the body, the red blood cells give up some of the air to the cells. Thus each cell of the body gets some air, and so it breathes. The cells cannot reach the air themselves, and so the red blood cells bring it to them. We breathe so as to supply the cells with air.

=105. What burning is.=--When meat is put into a hot stove it quickly burns, and passes off in smoke, and leaves only a little ashes. The ashes are the mineral parts of the meat. If the fire is very hot, you cannot see the smoke. The burning of the meat makes heat. Heat in a steam engine makes the machine do work.

Every fire must have plenty of air. If air is shut off, the fire goes out. When meat burns, the air unites with the meat and makes smoke, and ashes, and gives out heat. Air unites with something in every fire.

=106. Burning inside the body.=--In every part of a man's body a very slow fire is always burning. The blood brings to the cells food from the intestine, and air from the lungs. The food and air join in a burning. The smoke goes back to the blood and is carried to the lungs, and breathed out with the breath. The ashes, also, go back to the blood, and are carried away by the skin and kidneys. The burning makes no flame or light for it goes on very slowly. You cannot see the smoke, but you can feel the warmth of the burning. Some of the heat is turned to power, and gives the body strength to do work. The body is like a steam engine. It burns up all its food.

=107. How the body is warmed.=--The body is warmed by the slow burning in the cells. This burning keeps the body always at the same warmth. On a hot summer's day you feel warmer than on a cold snowy morning. But your body is no warmer. Only your skin is warmer.

If the skin is warm, the whole body feels warm, but if the skin is cold, the whole body feels cold. On a hot summer's day the heat is kept in the skin, and we feel warm. On a cold winter's day a great deal of heat passes off from the skin, and we feel cold. Yet our bodies have the same warmth in winter as in summer.

=108. How the sweat keeps us cool.=--When your hands or feet are wet, they are cold. On a hot summer's day, your body becomes wet with sweat. This cools the body as if water were poured over it. So sweating keeps you from getting too warm, and from being sunstruck.

We are sweating all the time, but the sweat usually dries as fast as it forms. When we are too warm it comes out faster than it dries. On a winter's day we sweat only a little, and so we save the heat. But more heat passes off from the skin into the cold air, and we do not grow warmer.

=109. Clothes.=--We wear clothes to keep the heat in the body. They do not make heat, but they keep it from going off. Wool and flannel clothes keep the heat in better than cotton. We wear woolen in the winter, and cotton in the summer.

Fur keeps in heat the best of all. In very cold lands only fur is worn.

Linen lets heat out easily. It makes good summer clothes.

=110. Where to wear the most clothes.=--The face and hands are kept warm by the blood and we do not cover them except in the coldest weather. Our feet are more tender and need to be covered enough to keep them warm. We ought to wear thick-soled shoes or rubbers in damp weather so as to keep the feet dry and warm. We ought to dry the stockings every night, for they will get wet with sweat.

The trunk of the body needs the most clothes. The legs ought to be kept warm, too. If the dress reaches only to the knee, thick underclothing is needed for the lower part of the leg.

Do not keep one part of the body warm while another part remains cold. It is wrong to bundle the neck or wear too much clothing over any part of the body. It is also wrong to wear too little and be cold.

When you are moving about, you need less clothing than when you are sitting still. When you have worked until you are very warm, it is wrong to stop to cool off. When you stop, you ought to put on a thick coat or else go into the house. If you do not, you may be chilled and made weak so that you can easily catch cold or some other disease.

=111. Heating houses.=--In winter our bodies cannot make heat fast enough to keep us warm unless we put on a great deal of clothing. So we warm our houses. Our grandfathers used fireplaces, but these did not give out much heat. People now use stoves, but some use a furnace in the cellar, or heat the rooms by steam. Some use kerosene stoves, but they are not so good, for they make the air bad. A room should feel neither too warm nor too cold. It is of the right warmth when we do not notice either heat or cold.

=112. Change of air.=--After air has been breathed it is no longer fit for use. In an hour or two you would breathe all the air of a small room once if it were not changed. When the air is partly used, you feel dull and short of breath, and your head aches. As soon as you get out of doors, you feel better. Foul air of houses and meeting places often contains disease germs. It is necessary to change the air of all rooms often. You can do this by opening a door or window. It is a good plan to sleep with your bedroom window open, so as to get good air all night.

Air passes in and out of every crack in the windows and doors. If only one person is in a room, this may make enough change of air. If many persons are in a room, you will need to change the air in other ways. You can do this by opening a door or window. Do not let the cold air blow upon any one, for it may help to make him catch cold, if the air of the room is impure. If we lower a window from the top, warm impure air may pass out above it without making a draft.

You need fresh air at night as much as in the daytime. You need not be afraid of the night air, for it is good and pure like the day air. You ought to sleep with your window open a little. You ought to open the windows wide every morning and air your bed well. At night you ought to take off all your clothes and put on a night-dress. Then hang your clothes up to air and dry.

=113. When to air a room.=--When you first enter a room full of bad air it smells musty and unpleasant. But after you have been in the room a while, you get used to it. If, however, you go out of doors a minute and then come back, you will smell the bad air again. If the air smells bad, open a door or window until it is sweet again.

=114. How to breathe.=--When you run hard, the cells of your body use up all the air, and then you feel short of breath. While you run, burning goes on faster, and you feel warmer. You can work harder and longer if you can breathe in a great deal of air. You will also feel better and stronger for it. Then if you are sick, you will be able to get well more quickly. You ought to know how to breathe right.

First, you ought to breathe through your nose. Even when you run, you ought to keep your mouth closed.

Second, you should try to breathe deeply. You should take a very deep breath often, and hold it as long as you can. By practice you can learn to hold it a full minute.

Third, you ought to run, or do some hard work, every day. When you get short of breath, you will have to breathe more deeply. After a while you may be able to run a half mile, or even a mile, without getting out of breath. But do not get tired out in your run, for this will harm you.

Fourth, you must sit and stand with your shoulders back, and your chest thrown forward. A round-shouldered boy cannot have large lungs or be long winded.

By breathing right, you can make your lungs very much larger and stronger.

=115. The voice.=--We talk by means of the breath. At the upper part of the windpipe is a small box. Its front corner can be felt in the neck, just under the chin, and is called the Adam's apple. Two thin, strong covers slide across the top of the box, and can be made to meet in the middle. The covers have sharp edges. When they are near together, and air is breathed out between them, a sound is made. This sound is the voice. The tongue and lips change it to form words.

=116. Care of the voice.=--The voice shows our feelings, even if we do not tell them in words. We can form a habit of speaking in a loud and harsh tone, as if we were always angry, or we can speak gently and kindly. We shall be more pleasant company to others if we are careful always to speak in gentle but distinct tones.

Shouting strains the voice and spoils its tone for singing. Reading until the throat is tired makes the voice weak. Singing or shouting in a cold or damp air is also bad for the voice. Breathing through the mouth is the worst of all for the voice.

=117. What becomes of alcohol in the body.=--When alcohol is taken up by the blood, it is carried to the liver. The liver tries to get rid of it by taking some air from the blood and burning it up, just as it burns the real food of the body. But this takes some air from the cells of the body. Then they do not burn as they should.

When a stove gets too little air through its draft, it makes an unpleasant smoke, and cools off. Just so, when the cells of the body do not burn as they should, they produce the wrong kind of smoke and ashes. This poisons the body and makes men sick. The most of the poisoning of alcohol is due to these new poisons.

When alcohol takes air from the cells of the body, they do not get enough air. Then they are like a short-winded boy, and do not do their work well. In this way alcohol makes the body weak.

Alcohol does not cease to be harmful because it is burned up in the body. It is harmful just because it burns so quickly. Using alcohol in the body is like trying to burn kerosene in a coal stove. The body is not made to burn alcohol any more than a coal stove is made to burn kerosene. You can burn a little kerosene in a coal stove if you are very careful. Just so, men can burn alcohol in their bodies. But kerosene will always smoke and clog up the stove, and may explode and kill some one. So alcohol in the body burns quickly and forms poisons. It always harms the body and may destroy life at once.

=118. Alcohol and the lungs.=--If you run a long race, your lungs will need a great deal of air. If you take strong drink, the alcohol will use up much of the air, and you will not have enough to use on your run. So you will feel short of breath, and will surely lose the race. You cannot drink and be long-winded.

Two drinks of whisky will use up as much air as the body uses in an hour. It would be easy to smother a person with strong drink. Drunken persons are really smothered; they often die because of the failure of their breathing, even while their heart is able to beat well.

Alcohol often causes the lungs to become thickened. Then air cannot easily pass through their sides, and a person suffers from shortness of breath. Sometimes these persons cannot lie down at all, but must sit up to catch their breath.

=119. Drinking and taking cold.=--A strong, healthy man can stand a great deal of cold and wet. If he breathes deeply in his work, all the cells of his body get plenty of air, and if he eats good food, the cells get plenty to eat. Then it will take a great deal to harm them. But alcohol hinders the digestion of their food, and also takes away their air. So the cells are both starved and smothered, and are easily hurt. Then a little cold and wet may do great harm to his body, for a drinker cannot stand bad weather or hard work so well as he could if he should leave drink alone.

Men often drink to keep themselves from taking cold. The alcohol really makes them more liable to take cold. It causes the blood to flow near the surface of the skin; there it is easily cooled, and the drinker soon becomes chilled; then he feels colder than ever. The cold harms the cells of his body, and then the white blood cells cannot easily fight disease germs. For this reason a drinker easily takes cold and other diseases.

=120. Alcohol lessens the warmth of the body.=--Alcohol causes the blood tubes in the skin to become larger. Then more blood will touch the cool air, and the body will become cooler. But because more warm blood flows through the skin, a man feels warmer. But he is really colder. Alcohol makes men less able to stand the cold. Travelers in cold lands know this and do not use it.

=121. How tobacco affects breathing.=--We would not live in a room with a smoking stove. But tobacco smoke is more harmful than smoke from a stove, for it has nicotine in it. Tobacco smoke in a room may make a child sick.

Cigarette smoking is very harmful to the lungs, for the smoke is drawn deeply into them, and more of the poison is likely to stay in the body. The smoke of tobacco burns the throat and causes a cough. This harms the voice.

WHAT WE HAVE LEARNED

1. Air is always being breathed into little sacs inside the body. The sacs form the lungs.

2. The red blood cells pass through the lungs, and take little loads of air. They then carry the air through the arteries to the capillaries.

3. In the capillaries the air leaves the red blood cells, and goes to the cells of the body.

4. The air unites with the cells, and slowly burns them to smoke and ashes.

5. The smoke goes back to the blood, and is carried to the lungs and given off by the breath. The ashes go back to the blood and pass off through the skin and the kidneys.

6. The burning in the cells makes heat.

7. Some of the heat is changed to power, as it is in a steam engine.

8. The heat also warms the body. It keeps it at the same warmth on a cold

day as on a hot day.

9. We wear clothes to keep the heat in, and so to keep us warm.

10. The air of a room needs to be changed often. It is made stuffy by our breath.

11. The voice is made by the breath in a box in the neck.

12. Alcohol uses air belonging to the cells of the body.

13. Tobacco smoke has the same poisons as tobacco. It can poison the whole body through the lungs.

CHAPTER XI

THE SKIN AND KIDNEYS

=122. Waste matters.=--The food is burned in the cells. As this burning goes on, the smoke goes off by the lungs and the unburned substances, the ashes, go off by the skin and kidneys. The ashes are mostly the minerals of the cells, but there are also some from the burned albumin. All these go back to the blood and are carried to the skin and kidneys.

=123. The skin.=--The skin covers the whole body. It is strong and keeps the body from being hurt.

=124. The epithelium.=--The skin is covered with a thin layer of cells like fine scales. These scales are called epithelium, or epidermis. They have no blood tubes or nerves and so have no feeling. You can run a pin under them without feeling pain. They are always growing on their under side and wearing off on their upper side. They keep the nerves and blood tubes of the skin from being hurt.

=125. The nails.=--The top scales of epithelium at the ends of the fingers become matted together to make the nails. The nails keep the ends of the fingers from being hurt. They can also be used to hold or cut small things. The new parts of the nails form under the skin and push down the older parts. So the nail grows farther than the end of the finger and needs to be cut off. Biting the nails leaves their ends rough. Then they may catch in the clothes and tear into the tender flesh. We ought to keep the nails cut even with the ends of the fingers.

The nails are not poisonous, but the dirt under them may be. We ought to keep them clean. Clean nails are one mark of a careful boy or girl.

=126. Hair.=--Some of the scales of epithelium over some parts of the body dip into tiny holes in the skin. In each hole they become matted together to form a hair. Fine short hair grows on almost every part of the body. On the top of the head it grows long and thick. When boys become men, it also grows long upon their faces. The skin pours out a kind of oil to keep the hair soft and glossy.

=127. Care of the hair.=--The hair may become dirty like any other part of the body. Brushing it takes out a great deal of dirt, but you should also wash it once a week.

The oil in the skin ought to be enough for the hair. Hair oils do not do the hair any good. If you wet the hair too often, you may make it stiff and take away its gloss. It is best to comb the hair dry. Brush it so as to spread the oil of the skin. Hair dyes are poisonous, and ought not to be used.

=128. The sweat or perspiration.=--The scales of epithelium dip into the skin and there line tiny tubes. The tubes form the sweat, or perspiration, out of the blood. The tubes are too fine to be seen, but they are upon almost every part of the body. They take the ashes or other waste matter or poisons from the blood and wash them out of the tubes with the perspiration. So the perspiration has two uses. First, it takes heat away from the body (see ?108).

Second, it gets rid of the waste matters or ashes of the body. It has very little of these at any one time, but in a day it gets rid of a great deal.

=129. The kidneys.=--The kidneys are close to the backbone, below the heart. They are made of tiny tubes much like the sweat tubes in the skin. The tubes take ashes and other waste matters from the blood, also a great deal of water. They also take away poisons and disease germs when we are sick. The kidneys take away about as much water as the skin, but they get rid of very much more poisons and waste matters than the skin does. If our kidneys should stop their work, we should soon die.

=130. Need of bathing.=--When the perspiration dries from the skin, it leaves the waste and poisons behind. We cannot always see the dried matters, but they always have an unpleasant odor. We should bathe often enough to keep our body from having an unpleasant smell. We should wash the whole body with soap and hot water at least once a week in winter and more often than that in summer.

Another reason for bathing is to wash disease germs from the body. Most dirt has disease germs in it. Disease germs also float in the dust of the air and stick to our skin when we go into a dusty room. If our skin is dirty, some of the germs may be carried into our flesh when our skin is pricked, or scratched, or cut. We sometimes catch boils, or erysipelas, or lockjaw, from very little wounds in a dirty skin. Cleanliness of our skin helps to keep us from catching diseases.

=131. Cold baths.=--Sometimes we bathe when we are clean so as to get refreshed. If we bathe in cold water, we feel cold at first. In a little while we feel warm again. Then we feel stronger, and refreshed for work. If we stay in the bath too long, we become cold again and feel weak. When boys go in swimming, they ought to come out before they begin to feel cold.

It is a good plan to take a cold bath every morning when you get up, even if you use only a wash-bowl with a little water. It will take only a few minutes, but will keep you clean and make you feel more like doing your day's work.

=132. A fair skin.=--We must wash often, to make the skin fair and smooth. Use enough good soap to keep the skin clean.

If you eat as you should, and digest the food well, your skin will have the least amount of waste to give off. Then it will look well. A bad looking skin is due to bad food and to bad digestion. If you do not digest your food well, you cannot have a fair skin.

Face paint and powder make the skin look worse, for they hinder perspiration. Nothing of that sort will do the skin any good. You must eat as you should, and you must keep clean. Then your skin will be clear.

=133. Washing clothes.=--Our clothes rub off a great deal of the perspiration and waste. They become soiled. A great deal of dirt also gets upon the sheets of our beds. Our clothes need to be washed as well as our bodies when they are soiled. Air and the sun as well as water destroy the waste of the body. Our clothes need to be aired at night, and the bed and bedroom should be aired through the day.

=134. Slops.=--After water has been used to wash our body or our clothes it is dirty and is not fit to be used again. It must not be thrown where it can run into a well. If a person has typhoid fever or cholera or other catching disease, the water may carry germs of the disease to the well, and so other persons may get it. Slops from the house should not be poured out at the back door, but they should be carried away from the house. In cities the slops are poured into large pipes and tunnels underground. These pipes are called sewers. They empty outside the city.

=135. Alcohol and the skin.=--Alcohol interferes with digestion and causes biliousness. This makes the skin rough and pimply. A drinker seldom has a clear skin.

Alcohol causes the arteries of the face to become enlarged. Then the face is red. A red nose is one of the signs of drinking. When a person uses strong drink he is often uncleanly. He does not care for the bad looks of his clothes and skin, and so he lets them stay dirty. This harms the skin and makes it look bad. The dirt also poisons the skin and may itself be a cause of sickness.

Because alcohol poisons the whole body and often produces kidney diseases, the drinker is apt to catch other diseases. Drinkers are the first to catch such diseases as smallpox and yellow fever. Where there are great numbers of cases, the drinkers are the first and often the only persons to die. This is because their skin and kidneys have been harmed by the alcohol and cannot throw off the poisons of the disease. Any kind of sickness will be worse in a drinker. Surgeons do not like to operate on drinkers, for their wounds do not heal so quickly as in other people.

When there is too little air, a fire burns slower, and makes a blacker smoke and more ashes. Alcohol takes some air from the cells of the body. So they burn with smoke and ashes of the wrong kind. The skin has to work harder to get rid of these, and sometimes it cannot do it well. Then the body is poisoned. The alcohol is burned and cannot poison the body any more. But it causes the body to make poisons, and so it is to blame. The poisons do great harm to the skin and kidneys. Alcohol causes more kidney disease than all other things put together.

WHAT WE HAVE LEARNED

1. Little tubes in the skin are always giving off ashes and waste matters in the perspiration.

2. Perspiration dries on the skin. So the skin must be washed often.

3. The kidneys get rid of more water and waste matter than the skin does.

4. Perspiration also gets upon the clothes and bed sheets. These must be

washed too.

5. Dirty water from washing should be thrown out where it cannot run into a well.

6. The skin is thick and strong and keeps the body from being hurt.

7. The skin is covered with a layer of scales. The scales have no feeling.

8. The scales form the nails on the ends of the fingers.

9. The scales also form the hair.

CHAPTER XII

THE NERVES, SPINAL CORD, AND BRAIN

=136. Need of nerves.=--The cells of the mouth, stomach, and intestine digest food; the cells of the liver change the food to blood; the cells of the heart pump the blood to feed all the cells of the body; the red blood cells carry air for the cells to breathe; and the cells of the skin and kidneys carry away the waste of the rest of the cells. Each set of cells works for all the rest. If the cells of the body were only tied together, each one would do as it pleased, and no two would work together. But something tells each cell of the body to work with the others. The cells all obey the mind. A tiny thread goes to each cell of the body. Each thread is a nerve. The mind and the cells signal to each other over the nerves. By means of the nerves the mind makes the cells work together.

=137. Nerve messages.=--The nerve threads run in bundles and form nerves large enough to be seen. The mind uses the nerves to tell the cells to do work. It tells the muscles to move the arms and legs. It tells the heart to beat and stomach to pour out gastric juice; and it tells each of the cells to eat.

The cells also send word over the nerves to the mind. They tell the mind when they are touching anything, and whether it is hard, or smooth, or hot, and many other things about it. The cells also tell the mind if they need more food, or are tired.

The nerves are always carrying messages to and from the cells. The cells depend upon these messages to tell them when and how to work. If the nerve of any part of the body is hurt or cut, we cannot feel with the part or move it, and its cells do not act in the right way. We do not feel the nerves while they are carrying the messages. We wish the cells of the arm to work, and they work, but we do not feel the message as it goes from the mind to the cells of the arm.

=138. The spinal cord.=--The nerves start inside the backbone. The backbone is hollow. It has a soft, white cord inside, as thick as the little finger. Part of the mind lives in this cord. The cord is called the spinal cord. Some of the nerves start from cells of the spinal cord. These cells send word to the muscles to move and to all the cells of the body to eat and grow. They also send word to the arteries to carry the right amount of blood to the cells.

From the nerves the spinal cord gets word when something hurts any part of the body. You may put your finger on a sharp pin. The spinal cord feels the prick, and quickly sends word to snatch the finger away. So the finger is taken away before you really feel the prick. When some one sticks a pin into you, you cannot help jumping. This is because the spinal cord sends word for you to jump away from the pin before it can harm you much. Thus the spinal cord keeps the body from being hurt. It acts while we are asleep as well as when we are awake.

=139. Need of a spinal cord.=--We do not feel the spinal cord acting, and we cannot keep it from acting. It tells the cells when to eat and grow, and it tells the heart and arteries how much blood to send to each cell. If we had to think about feeding an arm or a leg, we should sometimes forget it, but the spinal cord keeps doing it without our thinking of it. We put food into the body, and the spinal cord tells the cells to use it. If it stops acting for an instant, the cells stop work and we die. We cannot change its action by any amount of thinking.

=140. The brain.=--The nerves of the body go to the brain as well as to the spinal cord. The brain lies in the top of the head. A hard cover of bone keeps it from getting hurt. It is a soft white mass, and weighs about three pounds. Its outside is made of cells, while its inside is the very beginning of the nerves of the body.

=141. The mind.=--The mind is the real man. It is the thinking part of himself. It lives in the body and works by means of the cells of the brain. If these cells are hurt or killed, the body seems to have no mind, but yet it may keep on living. If all the mind leaves the body, the body is dead.

By means of the mind we feel, and know, and think. The mind uses each part of the brain for only one kind of work.

=142. The senses.=--The cells of the body send word to the brain over the nerves. The eye tells of sight, the ear of sounds, the nose of odors, the mouth of tastes, and the skin of feelings. All these messages go to the back part of the brain. They tell the mind of the news outside of the body. We get all our knowledge in this way. The cells also tell of their need of food and drink by means of the feelings of hunger and thirst.

=143. Motion.=--The mind in the cells of the top part of the head sends the orders for moving the different parts of the body. When we wish to run, the mind in the top of our head sends an order over our nerves to our legs, and they carry the body where we wish. If the top part of your brain is hurt, as by a blow, it cannot send orders to move, but you will lie stunned.

=144. Memory.=--The mind lays away all its messages, and often looks them over again. These old messages are called memories. They always stay with the brain, and the mind can call them up at any time. Our memories make our knowledge.

Every act of the mind leaves some mark on the memory. We may not be able to bring it back when we want to, but it will come back some time. Every bad word and evil deed will tend to come back and make us bad again. Every good work and word will leave its memory and make us better. We ought to fill our minds with good memories.

=145. Thinking.=--The brain also thinks. Thinking is different from feeling and from moving, but we can think about our feelings and about our movements. The brain just back of the forehead does all our thinking. A dog has only a little forehead, and cannot think much. But the rest of its brain is large, for it can see and hear and run as well as a man. A baby can see and hear and move, but it cannot think until it is taught how. Boys and girls go to school to learn to think. Thinking is work, just as truly as running is work. At school, no one can learn to think without working. Looking at things and hearing some one talk about them will not make you a strong-minded man, but thinking about these things will. Boys and girls should study and think, as well as look around and listen.

=146. How thought rules the body.=--We are always feeling and moving. We often do these things without trying, but we must make ourselves think. We can make our bodies move, or keep still, and we can keep from too much feeling. Our thoughts direct our natural desires to move and feel. In an animal, the feelings and movements direct the thoughts. When men let their feelings rule their thoughts, they are like animals. When the thoughts control the feelings and acts, we are men. If you get angry and cry, when you hurt your finger, then you are like an animal; but if you think about it and control your feelings, you are behaving like a strong and noble man. The thought part of the brain ought to rule all the rest.

=147. Sleep.=--Most of the brain does its work without our knowing it, but we know when we think. The thinking part of the brain gets tired, like any other part of the body. When it stops work, we are asleep.

We must give the brain a rest in sleep, just as we must rest an arm or a leg. We ought to give it regular rest. Every night we ought to go to bed early. Then we shall be ready to get up early and shall feel like working. Boys and girls need nine or ten hours' sleep each day. When they are grown, they need seven or eight hours' sleep each day.

The spinal cord and some parts of the brain must always stay awake to make the cells of the body eat and grow. When we are asleep, they must be wide awake, and must repair the worn-out parts. They do not seem to rest at all. If they rested for any length of time, then the lungs, heart, stomach and all other parts of the body would stop work, and we should die. But they really rest a part of the time. Like the heart, they act for a second, and then stop for a second. They seem to act all the time, but in all they rest half the time.

=148. Worry.=--The mind can do a great deal of work, if it gets good sleep. If a person gets enough sleep and rest, he cannot harm his mind by hard work. Sometimes the mind is troubled and worried over a danger or a loss. Then it cannot rest, but soon wears itself out. Worry is far more tiresome than hard work. By an effort, we can keep from worrying. It never does us good to worry, and we ought to keep from it.

=149. Nervousness.=--The thoughts are able to rule all the rest of the mind. They can keep us from feeling ill-tempered when we cannot have our own way. Sometimes a little unpleasant feeling makes us very unhappy, and keeps us from thinking about our work. A little noise or pain keeps some children from study, while others can bear a great deal without being disturbed by it. Some persons jump at a little noise, and are afraid of a tiny bug or mouse. This is because their feelings rule their thoughts. Such persons are called nervous.

A nervous person is very uncomfortable and makes others so too. Yet any one can get over the habit of being nervous, if he will try. You ought not to laugh at a nervous person if he is afraid of some little thing while you are not. You should help him to get over his nervousness and to become brave.

=150. Fear.=--Some persons are always brave. In danger they calmly stop to think, and then know how to save themselves. A timid person does not think, but rushes where his feelings lead. When a crowd is in danger, all will rush to do one thing. All will run for a door, and perhaps tread on one another. Then some one will surely be hurt. At a fire, or in any other danger, you should always stop to think how to act. If you rush with the crowd, you may be hurt. You will be more likely to be safe, if you stay away from them. Then, if help comes, you will be able to receive it. Besides, if you are cool and brave, you will help others around you to be brave too.

=151. Fire drill.=--In schools the children are taught how to go out of the building when there is a fire. A bell is struck when the children do not expect it. Then every child must leave his seat at once and march out of the building. The bell is struck every few days. Then, when the bell really sounds for a fire, the children know how to march out quickly, and so they learn to be brave.

By training we can learn to be brave at all times. We fear many harmless things, and in many cases do not fear real dangers. We are liable to be hurt at any time. We are more liable to be hurt by a horse when we are out driving than we are by the dark. Yet we do not fear the horse, while some do fear the dark. We ought to learn to think, so as to control our fear.

Some are afraid of the dark, some are frightened by ghost stories, and others expect to see a wild animal jump from behind every bush. No one fears these things unless he has been told about them. We ought to be careful not to tell children of these things. We ought to teach them to control their fear.

=152. Habit.=--After we have thought about a thing a few times, its hold on our memory becomes strong, and leads us to think about it often. When we have done a thing a few times, we are likely to do it again without knowing it. We call this doing things over again habit. When we once form a habit, we find it very hard to break. We can form habits of doing right or of doing wrong. We can get into the habit of swearing or of drinking by doing these things a few times. Then we shall do these things when we do not want to. When a drinker begins, he does not expect to keep on drinking. But his habit makes him drink, and he cannot help it. We should be careful not to do bad things, for we easily form the habit of doing them.

=153. Good habits.=--We can form habits of doing right. We can speak kindly and be generous. Then we shall do these things as easily as others get cross. After a person has tried to do good a few times, he will find it much easier to do good. Then he will speak kindly and give generously just as easily as others get angry and keep their good things to themselves.

=154. Alcohol takes away thought.=--Alcohol affects and weakens the cells of the brain sooner than it does those of any other part of the body. It first makes the thought cells weak. Then a person does not think how he acts. He lights his pipe in the barn and throws the match in the hay. He drives his horse on a run through a crowded street. He swears and uses bad language. He gets angry at little things and wants to fight. He seems to think of himself, and of no one else. He is happy, for he does not think of the bad effects of the drink. He has a good time, and does not care for its cost. He likes to drink, because it makes him feel happy.

=155. Alcohol spoils motion.=--Some cells of the brain cause the arms and legs, and all other parts of the body, to move. Alcohol next makes these weak. Then a person cannot move his legs right, but he staggers when he walks. He cannot carry a full cup to his lips. His hands tremble, and he cannot take care of himself. He is now really drunk.

=156. Alcohol takes away feeling.=--After a man is drunk, he loses the sense of feeling. He does not feel cuts and blows. Because he does not feel tired, he feels very strong. He often sees two things for one, and hears strange noises. The whole brain at last gets weak, and cannot act. Then the drinker lies down in a drunken sleep, and cannot be waked up. Some die in this state.

=157. Insanity.=--When the brain is misused by alcohol for some time, it cannot get over it. Then the person becomes insane. Drink sends more persons to the insane asylum than all other causes put together.

=158. Delirium tremens.=--If a drinker gets hurt, or becomes sick, he sometimes has terrible dreams. In them he sees dirty and savage animals coming to harm him. These dreams seem very real to him, and he cries out in his fright. This is called delirium tremens. A person is liable to die from it.

=159. Alcohol harms a drinker's children.=--The children of drinkers are apt to be weak in body and mind. A drinker hurts his children even more than he hurts himself. They are liable to catch diseases, and are often cross and nervous, or weak-minded. It is a terrible thing for a man to make his children weak and nervous.

=160. Other bad things about drink.=--There are many other terrible things about drink, besides the harm it does a man's body. Many a man has made himself drunk so as to steal or kill. No man can drink long without becoming a worse man for it. Men will not trust him, and he loses the respect of his friends.

Making strong drink takes thousands of men away from good work. They might work at building houses, or raising grain, or teaching school. As it is, their work is wasted.

A great deal of money is wasted on strong drink. All the mines of the world cannot produce enough gold and silver to pay the drink bill. The people of the United States pay more for strong drink than for bread.

The price of two or three drinks a day would amount to enough, in ten years, to buy a small home.

The cost of strong drink is made much greater if we count the cost of jails and insane asylums. Over one half of all crimes and cases of insanity are caused by strong drink.

We must also add the misery and suffering of most children of drunken fathers. This loss cannot be counted in money. Numbers of children become truants from school and learn theft and falsehoods from lack of a father's care. When all the cost is counted, nothing will be found so expensive as strong drink.

On the other hand, what do people get for their money and suffering? They get only a little pleasure, and then they are ashamed of it. Men use strong drink only because they like it more than they dislike its bad effects.

Since drink does a great deal of harm, with no good to any one, it is right to make laws to control its sale.

=161. How tobacco affects the brain.=--Some men smoke to make themselves think, and some to keep themselves from thinking. Now, smoking cannot do both things. It really makes the brain less able to think, for it weakens the whole body. A school-boy's brain will surely be harmed if he uses tobacco at all.

WHAT WE HAVE LEARNED

1. The mind makes all the cells of the body work together.

2. Tiny nerve threads carry messages from the mind to the cells.

3. Most of the nerves begin at the spinal cord in the backbone.

4. The mind in the spinal cord tells the cells to eat and grow. It tells the arteries how much blood to carry to the cells.

5. The cells tell the spinal cord if they need food, or if something suddenly hurts them. The spinal cord sends word to snatch the part from danger.

6. Nerves carry to the brain news of sight, sound, odor, taste, and touch.

7. The brain sends word to the muscles to move the arms, the legs, and the rest of the body.

8. The brain thinks.

9. The brain stores up all its messages; these make memory and knowledge.

10. The thought part of the brain can control the feelings and the movements of the body.

11. Alcohol is more harmful to the brain than to any other part of the body.

CHAPTER XIII

THE SENSES

=162.= A man has five ways of knowing about things outside of the body. He can feel, see, hear, smell, and taste.

=163. Feeling.=--Nerves go to nearly every cell in the body. They carry news to the brain when anything touches them. The news produces a feeling. Feelings are of three kinds:--

First, when anything touches the cells without harming them, we feel a touch. We feel a touch by nerves in the skin. Those in the ends of the fingers and tongue can feel the best. Those upon the back give but little feeling.

Touch tells whether anything is hard, or rough, or round, or square, or has other qualities and shapes.

Second, when anything touches the bare nerves or hurts the cells, we feel a pain. We can feel a pain anywhere in the body. Pain tells us if we are being harmed. If we had no feeling of pain, we might be killed before we could know of our danger. Pain warns us away from danger.

Third, we can feel heat and cold. Anything very hot or very cold, however, makes only a pain and gives no feeling either of cold or of heat.

=164. Sight.=--We see with our eyes. An eye is a hollow ball. In its front is a clear window. Behind the window is a round curtain with a round hole in its middle. When we speak of the color of the eye, we mean the color of this curtain. Light passes through the hole in the curtain and falls upon some nerves in the back of the eyeballs. There it forms a picture like a photograph. The nerves carry this picture to the brain, and we see it.

=165. Movements of the eyes.=--We can turn our eyes so as to look in any direction. Sometimes a person has one eye turned sidewise. Such a person is cross-eyed, and sees well out of only one eye at a time. Glasses may help the eyes, but sometimes a surgeon has to cut a tiny muscle.

=166. Coverings of the eyes.=--The eyeballs lie in a bony case, upon a soft bed of fat. In front each is covered with two lids. We can shut the lids to keep out dust and insects. When we are sleepy, they come together and cover the eyes. Little hairs at their edges help to keep out the dust.

Sometimes a little dirt gets under the lids. Then the eye smarts or itches, and we want to rub it; but this may grind the dirt in deeper. Then you should get some one else to lift your eyelid and pick out the dust with a soft handkerchief. If you cannot get help, lift the lid by the eyelashes; blow your nose hard, and the tears may wash the dirt away.

Dust and disease germs may get into our eyes and make them sore and red. You should bathe your eyes well every time you wash your face. You should use a clean towel, for a dirty one may carry disease germs to your eyes. Some forms of sore eyes are catching. If any one has sore eyes, no one else should use his towels or handkerchiefs.

=167. Tears.=--Clear salt water is always running over the eyes and down a tube into the nose. The use of this water is to bathe the eyes and keep them clean. It sometimes runs over the lids in drops called tears.

=168. How to use the eyes.=--If using your eyes makes them painful or gives you a headache, you are straining your eyes. Facing a bright light strains the eyes. Shade your eyes while you study. A cap may be used as a shade if you cannot get anything else. Never try to look at the sun or a very bright light. You should have the light at one side or behind you. The light should be steady. Reading in a dim light will harm the eyes.

=169. Near sight.=--If you cannot read without holding your book less than a foot from your eyes, you are nearsighted, and should wear glasses all the time. If you do this, your eyes may be strong, and you may be able to see well.

=170. Far sight.=--If you cannot read without holding your book at arm's length, you are farsighted and need glasses. Most old persons are farsighted.

=171. Alcohol and the eyes.=--Alcohol makes the eyes red. It weakens the eyes and may produce blindness. A drunken person often sees double.

=172. Tobacco= causes dimness of sight and sometimes produces blindness.

=173. Hearing.=--We hear with the ears. Sound is made by waves in the air. The part of the ear on the outside of the head catches the air waves and throws them inside the ear. These air waves strike against a little drum. Three little bones then carry the waves on to nerves farther inside the head. Animals can turn their ears and catch sound from any direction.

=174. Ear wax.=--Wax is formed just inside the ear. It keeps flies and insects from crawling into the ear. Boys in swimming sometimes get cold water into their ears. This may make them have an earache.

=175. How the throat affects the ear.=--An air tube runs from the inside of the ear to the mouth. Sometimes when you blow your nose, you blow air into the ear. This makes you partly deaf and you hear a roaring in your ears.

Sometimes when you have a cold in your throat, this little tube is stopped. Then your ear may ache and may even discharge matter. This may make you somewhat deaf. Earache and deafness are most often due to a cold in the throat and a stoppage of this tube.

Many little boys and girls are deaf and do not know it. They cannot hear the teacher well, and sometimes the teacher thinks they are bad or careless because they do not answer.

=176. Care of the ears.=--Very loud noises may harm the ear and make you deaf. When you expect a very loud noise, put your fingers in your ears to shut out the sound.

Boxing the ears may break their tiny drums and make you deaf.

Do not get cold water in your ear. This may cause an earache and make you deaf. If you get water in your ear while you are in swimming, turn your head to one side and shake it. This will get the water out.

Do not put cotton or anything else into your ears.

=177. Smell.=--We smell with the nose. Some things give out a vapor to the air. When we draw the air into the nose, this vapor touches the nerves, and we perceive a smell. The nerves are high up in the nose. In order to perceive smell clearly, we sniff the air far up the nose.

=178. Use of smell.=--Bad air and spoiled food smell bad. A bad smell is the sign of something spoiled. The sense of smell tells us when food or air is unfit for use. Some people try to hide a bad smell with perfumery. To do this only makes the danger greater, for then the smell does not tell us of the danger of food or air.

Some animals can smell much better than a man. A dog will smell the track of a wild animal hours after it is made. Savages can smell much better than civilized men.

=179. Taste.=--We taste with the tongue. Dry food has no taste, but it must first dissolve in the mouth. Spoiled food tastes bad. Bad-tasting food is not fit to eat. Taste tells us whether food is good or bad.

We can learn to like the taste of harmful things. At first no one likes tobacco or strong drink, but the liking is formed the more one uses these. We ought to be careful not to begin to use such things.

Alcohol and tobacco burn the mouth and harm the taste. Food does not taste so good and we may eat spoiled food and not know it.

WHAT WE HAVE LEARNED

1. We can feel in every part of the body, but mostly in the ends of the fingers.

2. Light makes a picture upon the nerves inside of the eye.

3. If the eyes ache, the light should be softened or the position of the book or work changed, or else the eyes should be rested.

4. Sound in the air goes into the ear and strikes against a drum. Bones then carry the sound to the ear nerves.

5. Air snuffed up the nose gives the sense of smell. Smell tells us if the air or food is fit for use.

6. Taste tells us whether food is fit for use. Men can learn to like the taste of wrong things like tobacco or alcohol.

CHAPTER XIV

BONES AND JOINTS

=180.= Bones make the body stiff and strong, and give it shape. Long bones reach through the arms and legs, and little bones reach down the fingers and toes. Rounded plates of bone form the head, and a pile of bony rings makes up the backbone. Each bone is built to fit exactly into its own place and to do its own work. In all there are over two hundred bones in the body. They form one seventh of its weight.

=181. Form of bones.=--A bone is not like a solid piece of timber, but is hollow like the frame of a bicycle. This makes it strong and light. At its ends a bone is like a hard sponge covered with a firm shell. This makes it too strong to be easily crushed, and keeps it light.

A bone grows like any other part of the body. It is made of living cells like woven threads. Lime is mixed among the cells, and makes them stiff like starch among the threads of a linen collar. Blood tubes go through every part of the bone so as to feed the cells. The living cells form one third of the bone, while the lime forms two thirds.

=182. Broken bones.=--Bones are very hard, and yet they can bend a little without breaking. Most of them are curved a little, and so they will spring instead of breaking when they are pressed hard. But sometimes they break. Then a person must wear a splint and bandage to keep the bones in place until they grow together again. The living cells will mend a bone in about a month.

An old person's bones are more tender than a child's, and will not spring much without breaking. An old man is afraid of falling and breaking his bones, while a child falls a dozen times a day without danger.

The bones of some children bend too easily. When they stand, the bones of their legs bend a little. After a while they grow in the crooked shape, and the child is bow-legged.

=183. Joints.=--Some bones are hinged upon each other. A bone hinge is a joint. The rings of the backbone are held together by very tough pads of flesh. Each pad lets the backbone bend only a little, but altogether they let us bend our backs in any direction. These pads are like rubber springs in a wagon, and keep our bodies from being jarred too much.

The finger and toe joints, the wrists and ankles, the elbows and the knees, bend back and forth like a hinge. Tough bands of flesh bind the bones together. The ends of the bones are rounded and smooth. They fit together and make perfect hinges. The joints are oiled by a fluid like the white of an egg. In old people this fluid sometimes dries up. Then the joints become stiff, and creak like a squeaking hinge.

[Illustration: =Hinge joint of the elbow.=

1 humerus 2 ulna]

The shoulders and hips can be moved in every direction. The upper ends of the arm and leg bones are round like half a ball. They fit into cups on the shoulder and hip bones. They are very smooth, and are oiled like the hinge joints. The joints are made to work very smoothly and easily.

=184. Bones out of joint.=--When the ends of bones are torn away from each other, the bone is out of joint. Then the bone cannot be moved without great pain. It should be put back in place at once and kept there by splints and bandages. A person is less liable to have his joints out of place than he is to have his bones broken.

=185. Sprains.=--Sometimes a joint is turned too much. This stretches the flesh around the joint, and makes it very tender and painful. This is a sprain. When you sprain a joint, you should put it in hot water for an hour or two. Then keep it still for a few days.

=186. Why bones and joints grow wrong.=--While bones and joints are growing they can be made to take any shape we please. They cannot be bent all at once, but if we hold them in one way much of the time, they will keep that shape. Some boys and girls sit with their backs bent forward and lean against the desk as if they were too lazy to sit up. When they grow up, they will be bent and round-shouldered. You should sit and stand straight. Then you will grow tall and straight and strong. A soldier has square shoulders and walks erect because he is drilled until his bones and joints grow in the proper shape. As you stand straight with your feet together, your two big toes, your two ankles, and your two knees should touch each other.

If you wear tight shoes and press the toes out of shape, they will soon grow so. Nearly every one's feet are out of shape from wearing short, pointed shoes. Your toes should be straight and not cramped by the shoe. If you wear narrow shoes, you may harm your feet. It is better to have one's feet useful, even if they are large, than to make them small and useless.

WHAT WE HAVE LEARNED

1. Bones make the body stiff, and give it form.

2. Some bones are long, some round, and some flat. All are hard and springy.

3. Some bones are hinged together. The hinge is a joint.

4. The ends of bones in joints are rounded and smooth, and are oiled with a liquid like the white of an egg.

5. Some bones are bound together by springy pads, as in the backbone.

6. Bones can be broken. They will grow together again themselves.

7. Joints can be put out of place; then we must put them back.

8. If joints or bones are kept in wrong positions they will grow into bad shapes. Tight shoes deform the feet.

CHAPTER XV

MUSCLES

=187. Shape of muscles.=--Bones are covered with muscles. Muscles give shape to the body, and move it about. One half of the body consists of muscles. These are arranged in bundles, and each causes a bone to make one motion. There are over four hundred separate bundles of muscle in the body.

One end of a muscle is large and round and is fast to a bone. The other end tapers to a strong string or tendon. The tendon passes over a joint, and becomes fast to another bone. You can easily feel the tendons in the wrist and behind the knee.

A muscle is made of tiny strings. You can pick them apart until they are too fine to be seen with the eye. Each string is a living muscle cell. It is the largest kind of cell in the body. You can see the fine strings in cooked meat.

=188. How muscles act.=--A nerve runs from the brain, and touches every cell of the muscle. When we wish to move, the brain sends an order down the nerve. Then each muscle cell makes itself thicker and shorter. This pulls its ends together, and bends the joint. We can make muscle cells move when we wish to, but we cannot make any other kind of cell move. We make all our movements by means of our muscles.

=189. Where you can see muscles.=--In a butcher's shop you can see lean meat. This is the animal's muscle. White and tough flesh divides the tender red meat into bundles. Each red bundle is a muscle. You will see how the muscle tapers to a string or tendon. The butcher often hangs up the meat by the tendons. You can see the muscles and tendons in a chicken's leg or wing when it is being dressed for dinner.

Roll up your sleeve to see your own muscles. Shut your hand tight. You will see little rolls under your skin, just below the elbow. Each roll is a muscle. You can feel them get hard when you shut your hand. You can feel their tendons as they cross the wrist.

Open your hand wide. You can see and feel the tendons of the fingers upon the back of the hand. These tendons come from muscles on the back of the arm. You can feel the bundles of these muscles when they open the fingers. There are no muscles in the fingers, but all are in the hand or arm. You cannot open your hand so strongly as you can close it.

=190. Strength of muscle.=--By using a muscle you can make it grow larger and stronger. If you do not use your muscles they will be small and weak. Children ought to use their muscles in some way, but if they use them too much, they will be tired out. Then they will grow weaker instead of stronger. Lifting heavy weights, or running long distances, tires out the muscles, and makes them weaker. Small boys sometimes try to lift as much as the big boys. This may do their muscles great harm.

=191. Round shoulders.=--The muscles hold up the back and head, and keep us straight when we sit or stand. A lazy boy will not use his muscles to hold himself up, but will lean against something. He will let his shoulders fall, and will sit down in a heap. Sometimes he is made to wear shoulder braces to keep his shoulders back. This gives the muscles nothing to do, and so they grow weaker than ever. The best thing to do for round shoulders is to make the boy sit and stand straight, like a soldier. Then he will use his muscles until they are strong enough to hold his shoulders back.

=192. How exercise makes the body healthy.=--When you use your muscles, you become warmer. Your face will be red, for the heart sends more blood to the working muscle cells. You will be short of breath, for the cells need more air. You will eat more, for your food is used up. Your muscles are like an engine. They get their power from burning food in their own cells. When they work they need to use more food and air. So working a muscle makes us eat more and breathe deeper. The blood flows faster, and we feel better all over. The muscle itself grows much larger and stronger.

If we sit still all day, the fires in our bodies burn low and get clogged with ashes. We feel dull and sleepy. If we run about for a few minutes, we shall breathe deeply. The fires will burn brighter. Our brains will be clearer, and we shall feel like work again. Boys and girls need to use their muscles when they go to school. Games and play will make you get your lessons sooner.

=193. How to use the muscles.=--You should use your muscles to make yourself healthy, and not for the sake of growing strong. Some very strong men are not well, and some men with small muscles are very healthy. Some boys have strong muscles because their fathers had strong muscles before them. Strength of muscle does not make a man.

You ought to have healthy muscles. Then your whole bodies will be healthy, and you can do a great deal of work. You ought to learn how to use your muscles rather than how to make them strong. An awkward and bashful boy may be very strong, but he cannot use his muscles. A boy is graceful because he can use them.

The best way to use your muscles is in doing something useful. You can help your mother in the house and your father at the barn. You can run errands. You can learn to use carpenter's tools or to plant a garden. Then you will get exercise and not know it. You will also be learning something useful.

Play is also needed. Work gets tiresome, and you will not want to use your muscles. Play is bad when it takes you from your work or when you hurt yourself trying to beat somebody.

=194. Alcohol and the muscles.=--Men use alcohol to make themselves strong. It dulls their weak feelings, and then they think themselves strong. They are really weaker. The alcohol hinders digestion and keeps food from the cells. Then the fires in the body burn low, and there is little strength.

Alcohol sometimes causes muscle cells to change to fat. This weakens the muscles.

Men sometimes have to do hard work in cold countries; and at other times they must make long marches across hot deserts. Neither the Eskimos in the cold north, nor the Arabs in the hot desert, use strong drink. Alcohol does not help a man in either place. It really weakens the body. The government used to give out liquor to its soldiers; but soldiers can do more work and have better health without liquor and it is no longer given out.

A few years ago men were ashamed to refuse to drink. Even when a new church building was raised, rum was bought by the church and given to the workmen. Farmers used to give their men a jug of rum when they went to work. Farm hands would not work without it.

Now all this has changed. Men do not want drinkers to work for them. A railroad company will discharge a man at once if he is known to drink at all. A man can now refuse to drink anywhere and men will not think any less of him.

=195. Tobacco= poisons the muscle cells and makes them weak. At first it makes boys too sick to move. It always poisons the cells even if they do not feel sick.

=196. A long life.=--A man's body is built to last eighty years, but only a few live so long. If you are careful in your eating and drinking, if you breathe pure air, and if you use your muscles, your body will be healthy and will last the eighty years and more. All through your life you will be strong and able to do good work.

WHAT WE HAVE LEARNED

1. Muscles cover the bones and move the body.

2. Muscle is lean meat. It is made of bundles of cells like strings. Nerves from the brain touch each cell.

3. Each muscle is fast to a bone. It becomes a small string or tendon at the other end. The tendon crosses a joint and is fast to another bone.

4. When we wish to move, the brain sends an order to the muscle cells to make themselves thicker and shorter and so bend the joint.

5. You can feel the muscles and tendons in the arm and wrist.

6. Muscle work makes us breathe deeper, and eat more food. It makes the blood flow faster. So it makes our whole bodies more healthy.

7. Every one ought to use his muscles some part of the day.

8. Alcohol and tobacco lessen the strength of the muscles.

CHAPTER XVI

DISEASE GERMS

=197. Catching diseases.=--Our body may get out of order like a machine. Some parts of it may be cut, or broken, or worn out, or hurt in other ways. Then we are sick until it is made whole again. Sickness always means that a part of the body is out of order.

Some kinds of sickness are like a fire. A small bit of something from a sick person may start a sickness in us, just as a spark may set a house on fire. Then we may give the sickness to others, just as a fire may spread to other houses. If a person has measles, we may catch the measles if we go near him; but if a person has a toothache, we cannot catch the toothache from him. So we may catch some kinds of diseases, but we cannot catch other kinds.

=198. Bacteria and germs.=--Every kind of catching sickness is caused by tiny living things growing in our flesh and blood. Some of them are tiny animals. Most of them are plants, and are called bacteria or microbes. A common name for all of them is germs.

The word germ means nearly the same as the word seed. Bacteria are so small that we cannot see them unless we look at them through a strong microscope. Then they look like little dots and lines (p. 54). A million of them could lie on a pin point; but if they have a chance, they may grow in numbers, so that in two days they would fill a pint measure.

Very many kinds of bacteria and other germs are found nearly everywhere. They are in the soil and in water, and some float in the air as dust. When they fall on dead things, they cause decay or rotting. When we can fruit, we kill the germs by boiling the fruit and the cans. Then we close the cans tightly so that no new germs can get into them. The fruit will then keep fresh for years.

Decay is nearly always a good thing, for by it dead bodies and waste substances are destroyed and given back to the ground, where plants feed upon them. Many plants would not grow if they could not feed upon decaying things. So most bacteria and other germs are useful to us. But some kinds of germs will grow only in our bodies, and these kinds are the cause of most of our sickness.

=199. Germs of sickness.=--We catch a sickness by taking a few of the germs of the sickness into our flesh. There they grow quickly, like weed seeds in the ground, and form crops of new germs within a few hours. After a few days the germs become millions in number, and crowd the cells of our flesh, just as weeds may crowd a potato plant (p. 54).

Disease germs in the body also form poisons, just as some weeds in a field form poisons. The poisons make us sick, just as if we had swallowed the leaves of a poisonous weed.

=200. Fever.=--If a sickness is caused by disease germs, the body is nearly always too warm. Then we say that the sick person has a fever. Almost the only cause for a fever is disease germs growing in the body. We can make a person have any kind of fever by planting a few of the germs of the fever in the right part of his body.

We are made sick by the germs of fevers more often than by all other causes put together. Here is a list of common diseases caused by fever germs:--colds and sore throats, most stomach aches, blood poisoning in wounds, boils and pimples, tuberculosis, whooping cough, measles, chicken pox, diphtheria, scarlet fever, typhoid fever, smallpox, and malaria.

Which of these kinds of sickness have you had? What sickness have you had besides these?

=201. Sickness and Dirt.=--Disease germs leave the body of a sick person in three ways: first, through the skin, second, through the kidneys and intestines, and third, through the nose and throat. In these same ways our body gives off its waste matters. If we did not take anything from another person's body into our own body we should not catch fevers.

Whatever a feverish person soils may contain disease germs. When a person has only a slight fever he often keeps at work, and then he may scatter disease germs wherever he goes. So disease germs are likely to be found wherever there is dirt or filth. Cleanliness means good health as well as good looks.

=202. Disease germs in the skin.=--Disease germs may often be found in sores and pimples on the skin, but they will not leave anybody's flesh and blood through sound and healthy skin. If our skin is smooth and fair, there will be few disease germs on it unless we rub against something dirty. A dirty skin nearly always contains disease germs. Washing and bathing our body will take disease germs from our skin and help us to keep well.

=203. Disease germs in slops.=--A great many disease germs leave the body through the intestine and kidneys, and may be found in the slops and waste water of our houses. Slops are dangerous to health, for they may run into a well, or spring, or river, and so carry disease germs into our drinking water (p. 27). Also, house flies may light on the pails or puddles and carry the germs to our food. In these ways we catch typhoid fever, stomach aches, and other diseases of the intestines. All slops and waste matters from the body should be put where they cannot reach our drinking water, and where flies cannot crawl over them (p. 80).

=204. Disease germs from the nose and throat.=--If a person is sick with a fever, many of the germs are likely to be found in his nose and throat. Thousands of them are driven out with every drop of saliva and phlegm when he blows his nose, or spits, coughs, or sneezes, or talks. If he puts anything into his mouth, it will be covered with germs. More diseases are spread from the nose and mouth than in any other way, for we are always doing something to spread bits of saliva and phlegm.

=205. Spitting.=--Colds and consumption and other forms of sickness are often spread by sick persons spitting on the floor or pavement. The germs become dried and are blown away as dust. For this reason dust from the streets of cities and in crowded halls is often the cause of sickness. In many places spitting on a floor or pavement is strictly forbidden by law.

=206. Putting things in the mouth.=--Many persons have the habit of sucking their fingers, or of touching a pencil to the tongue when they write or think, or of wetting their fingers with their lips when they turn the leaves of a book. In all these ways we may give a disease to others or may take a disease from some one else.

=207. Public drinking cup.=--When you touch your lips to a cup, you leave some saliva and cells from your mouth on the cup. If a cup is used by a number of persons, some one is almost sure to leave germs of sickness on it, and others are likely to take them into their own mouths when they drink. So a public drinking cup is a dangerous thing. Each school child should have his own cup. Public drinking fountains should be so made that we may drink by putting our lips to a stream of running water.

=208. Sweeping.=--Dusty air in a room is dangerous to health, for disease germs are likely to be found in it. We can get rid of dust by keeping our floors swept clean. After sweeping we should wipe the dust from the tables and furniture. A feather duster or dry cloth will only stir up the dust and make it float in the air again. We should use either a damp cloth, or a dry duster made of tufts of wool, so that the dust will stick to the duster.

=209. Foul air.=--If we live in a closed room, the air soon becomes foul and dusty, and is likely to have disease germs in it. Foul air is one of the greatest of the causes of sickness. We should change the air of a room often so as to keep it fresh and free from dust and disease germs (pp. 65-67).

=210. House flies.=--House flies come from garbage heaps and filth of all sorts. So they carry disease germs on their bodies. They light on our food and on our faces, and so they often make us sick. They are often the cause of typhoid fever, stomach aches, and stomach sickness in babies.

Flies are hatched in manure piles and garbage heaps. At first they look like white worms, and are called maggots. Every maggot is a young fly. We can get rid of flies by cleaning up every garbage heap and manure pile.

=211. Mosquitoes.=--Mosquitoes carry malaria and yellow fever from sick persons to the well. If there were no mosquitoes, there would be no malaria or yellow fever.

Mosquitoes are hatched in water, and the young are called wigglers. We may often see them in rain barrels. We may get rid of mosquitoes by emptying all rain barrels and pails and cans of dirty water, at least once a week, and by drying up swamps and marshes.

WHAT WE HAVE LEARNED

1. We catch a fever by taking disease germs into the body.

2. Disease germs cannot be seen without a strong microscope.

3. The germs may be found in dust and dirt.

4. Slops from our houses are often full of the germs.

5. You may take germs into your body by putting pencils and other things into your mouth, and by drinking from a public drinking cup.

6. Spitting on the floor or pavement may scatter disease germs.

7. House flies and mosquitoes often spread diseases.

CHAPTER XVII

PREVENTING SICKNESS

=212. How our body kills disease germs.=--We take disease germs into the body in three ways: first, through the mouth, second, through the nose, and third, through the skin. So we should watch the purity of our food, drink, and air, and should be careful about putting things into the mouth, and about the cleanliness of the skin. We often take a few disease germs into the body without catching a disease. This is because the white cells of our blood fight the germs and kill them (p. 53). If the body is hurt or weakened, the white blood cells may also be weakened so that they cannot kill the germs. We should take good care of the body so that every part of it may do its work well. We need not be able to run fast, or to lift heavy weights, but the best sign that every part of the body is in good order is to feel bright and wide-awake. Then our white blood cells will also be in good order and able to fight disease germs.

=213. Catching cold.=--When we catch a disease, we often say that we have caught cold. We used to think that cold air and dampness were almost the only causes of taking cold, and this is the reason why we called many kinds of sickness by the name of colds. Now we know that we catch cold by taking disease germs into the body. The germs will not be able to grow unless the body is weakened in some way, as by cold and dampness. Yet if we are wet and cold, we shall not catch cold unless we take disease germs into the body. We do not get the germs from the outdoor air, for very few germs are there. We get them from the foul air of our houses when we come in to warm and dry ourselves. If the air of our houses were always as clean and pure as the outdoor air, we should hardly ever have colds.

We can safely let the cold air blow on us if we are out of doors, but if we sit in a house, a small draft sometimes seems to make us take cold. This is because there are likely to be many disease germs in the house and few out of doors.

Other things besides cold air and dampness may weaken the body, and so help us to take cold. If germs of colds are in a warm room, we may sit there and take cold even if we are not wet or chilled at all. The body may be weakened by poor food, wrong eating, or overwork, so that disease germs will easily grow in it. We take as many colds from these causes as from cold air and dampness.

=214. Kinds of colds.=--A person takes most of the germs of colds through his nose and mouth. If they grow only in his nose, we say that he has a cold in his head. If they grow in his throat, he has a sore throat, or tonsillitis. If they reach as far as the upper part of his windpipe, he is hoarse, or has a cough, or the croup. If the germs are planted in his lungs, he may have bronchitis or pneumonia. All these kinds of sickness often spread from one person to another. If one person in a family has a cold, others in the family often catch cold from him.

=215. Diseases like colds.=--Diphtheria, tuberculosis, whooping cough, and measles all begin like a common cold and often look like a cold during the whole sickness. Colds do not turn into any of these diseases, for each of them comes from its own germ, just as corn comes only from seed corn.

=216. Curing a cold.=--If you have a cold, you ought to stay at home and rest, or lie in bed. Then your white blood cells can gain strength to fight the disease germs. You ought to have plenty of fresh air in your room. You ought not to eat much food for a few days, so that your stomach and intestine and liver can use all their strength in throwing off the poisons of the germs. But you ought to drink plenty of water, so as to help wash away the poisons from your body.

=217. Keeping colds from spreading.=--You should keep away from other persons while you have a cold, or other catching disease, so as to keep from spreading the sickness. You ought not to go visiting, or go to school, or to church, or to other meeting places. When you cough or sneeze, you should hold a handkerchief to your mouth, so as to keep from blowing disease germs from your throat and nose. You ought to sleep in a bed by yourself, so that no one may take the disease germs from your bedclothes. No one else should use your towel, or handkerchief, or knife, or fork, or spoon, or dish, until they have been washed in hot water, so as to kill the disease germs on them.

=218. Keeping from catching cold.=--You can keep yourself from catching cold by keeping your body strong and in good order. You should keep your clothes dry, eat good food, breathe pure air, get good rest and sleep, and keep your body, your clothes, and your house clean. You should also keep disease germs out of your body. You should not form a habit of putting your fingers or a pencil to your mouth (p. 127). You should keep your nose, your throat, and your mouth clean.

=219. Cleanliness of the nose.=--The inside of the nose is wet with a slippery liquid. If you have a cold, the liquid is thick and stops your nose, and is called phlegm. The liquid catches and holds dust and disease germs, and keeps them from going into the windpipe. It also kills many of the disease germs.

You should always carry a handkerchief and use it so as to blow the germs out of your nose. You should have a clean handkerchief every day.

[Illustration: =Photograph of model of the nose and throat.=

A. tonsil; B. adenoids; C. opening of Eustachian tube.]

=220. Adenoids and large tonsils.=--Sometimes children have large tonsils growing in the back of the throat, or soft bunches of flesh called adenoids back of the nose. These children cannot breathe well through the nose, but must breathe through the mouth. Then they take dust and disease germs deep into the body, and so take colds and other sickness easily. If a child has adenoids or large tonsils, an operation should be done to take them out.

=221. Cleanliness of the mouth.=--We often breathe dust and disease germs into the mouth or snuff them into the throat from the nose. Then they are caught between the teeth and in the folds of the cheeks and throat. There they may grow, and finally go deeper into the body and make us sick. A dirty mouth is very often the cause of colds and other sickness.

We should keep our mouths clean by brushing our teeth with a toothbrush two or three times a day. We should also rub the toothbrush over the tongue and around the back part of the throat so as to clean the germs from every part of the mouth. Each child should have a toothbrush of his own, and should use it every day.

=222. Contagious diseases.=--Diphtheria, whooping cough, measles, scarlet fever, and smallpox are all dangerous kinds of sickness, and spread with great ease. The germs may float in the air, and we may take them into our bodies if we go into a room where any one has the sickness. So we call these diseases contagious. If a person has one of these diseases, he should be made to stay in a house or room by himself until he is well. Keeping the sick away from well persons is called quarantine. When the sickness is cured, the sick room and everything in it should be cleaned and washed so as to kill the germs.

=223. Board of health.=--There is a board of health in every city and town. The men on the board show persons how to keep diseases from spreading, and make them obey the rules of health. Everybody in a town should help the board of health in every possible way.

WHAT WE HAVE LEARNED

1. The white blood cells of our body kill disease germs.

2. We catch cold by taking disease germs into our body.

3. The germs of colds are not often found in the air out of doors. They are often found in the foul air of houses.

4. If a person has a cold, he should keep away from other persons, so as to keep from spreading the sickness.

5. Cleansing the nose helps us to keep from catching cold.

6. Cleansing the teeth and the inside of the mouth removes many disease germs.

7. Adenoids and large tonsils should be taken from the throat by an operation.

8. If a person has a dangerous contagious disease, he should be quarantined.

9. Boards of health have charge of the prevention of contagious diseases.

###

www.ingramcontent.com/pod-product-compliance
Lightning Source LLC
Chambersburg PA
CBHW070231210526

45168CB00020B/2022